Clinically Oriented Theory
for Occupational Therapy

D1567123

Clinically Oriented Theory for Occupational Therapy

Christopher J. Alterio, DrOT, OTR

Assistant Professor of Occupational Therapy
Keuka College
Keuka Park, New York

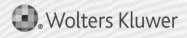

Philadelphia • Baltimore • New York • London
Buenos Aires • Hong Kong • Sydney • Tokyo

Executive Editor: Michael Nobel
Development Editor: Amy Millholen
Editorial Coordinator: Kerry McShane
Marketing Manager: Shauna Kelley
Production Project Manager: Barton Dudlick
Design Coordinator: Holly McLaughlin
Manufacturing Coordinator: Margie Orzech-Zeranko
Prepress Vendor: S4Carlisle Publishing Services

Copyright © 2019 Wolters Kluwer.

All rights reserved. This book is protected by copyright. No part of this book may be reproduced or transmitted in any form or by any means, including as photocopies or scanned-in or other electronic copies, or utilized by any information storage and retrieval system without written permission from the copyright owner, except for brief quotations embodied in critical articles and reviews. Materials appearing in this book prepared by individuals as part of their official duties as U.S. government employees are not covered by the above-mentioned copyright. To request permission, please contact Wolters Kluwer at Two Commerce Square, 2001 Market Street, Philadelphia, PA 19103, via email at permissions@lww.com, or via our website at lww.com (products and services).

9 8 7 6 5 4 3 2 1

Printed in China

Library of Congress Cataloging-in-Publication Data

Names: Alterio, C. J. (Christopher John), author.
Title: Clinically-oriented theory for occupational therapy / Christopher J.
   Alterio.
Description: Philadelphia: Wolters Kluwer Health, [2019] | Includes
   bibliographical references and index.
Identifiers: LCCN 2018027353 | ISBN 9781496389534 (paperback)
Subjects: | MESH: Occupational Therapy | Models, Theoretical | Clinical
   Medicine
Classification: LCC RM735.3 | NLM WB 555 | DDC 615.8/515—dc23 LC record available at
   https://lccn.loc.gov/2018027353

This work is provided "as is," and the publisher disclaims any and all warranties, express or implied, including any warranties as to accuracy, comprehensiveness, or currency of the content of this work.

This work is no substitute for individual patient assessment based upon healthcare professionals' examination of each patient and consideration of, among other things, age, weight, gender, current or prior medical conditions, medication history, laboratory data and other factors unique to the patient. The publisher does not provide medical advice or guidance and this work is merely a reference tool. Healthcare professionals, and not the publisher, are solely responsible for the use of this work including all medical judgments and for any resulting diagnosis and treatments.

Given continuous, rapid advances in medical science and health information, independent professional verification of medical diagnoses, indications, appropriate pharmaceutical selections and dosages, and treatment options should be made and healthcare professionals should consult a variety of sources. When prescribing medication, healthcare professionals are advised to consult the product information sheet (the manufacturer's package insert) accompanying each drug to verify, among other things, conditions of use, warnings and side effects and identify any changes in dosage schedule or contraindications, particularly if the medication to be administered is new, infrequently used or has a narrow therapeutic range. To the maximum extent permitted under applicable law, no responsibility is assumed by the publisher for any injury and/or damage to persons or property, as a matter of products liability, negligence law or otherwise, or from any reference to or use by any person of this work.

LWW.com

CCS0818

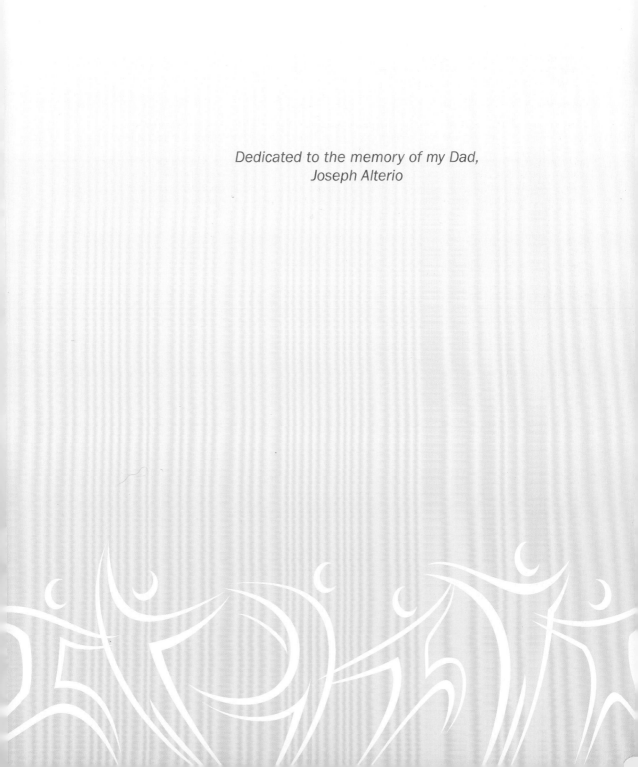

Dedicated to the memory of my Dad,
Joseph Alterio

Foreword

I have known Dr. Chris Alterio for many years, primarily through our work together on a variety of projects associated with the National Board for Certification in Occupational Therapy. I know him to be a clear thinker, a master clinician, and an exemplary educator. With this text, he has written one of the best and most informative textbooks on occupational therapy theory available today. This book is a must-read for students learning the basics of their chosen profession and for clinicians struggling to understand the myriad theoretical models on which they can base their practice. Educators will applaud this effort, which provides clear descriptions of past and current conceptual models for practice.

Dr. Alterio has undertaken the task of identifying prominent theoretical models and organizing them on the basis of paradigms and paradigm shifts throughout the history of the profession. He traces the historical roots, influences, and rationale for paradigm consensus and crisis, from the initial paradigm of occupation to medical model reductionism to paradigm crisis resolution.

He clearly advocates occupation-based approaches to practice, along with Reilly's NOBA principle, which acknowledges the importance of *not only* biomedical levels of concern *but also* biosocial levels of concern. The biomedical level provides valuable treatment methods associated with improving disabling conditions. The biosocial level provides occupation focus with treatment methods targeted at improving play, work, skill development, productive participation, and social engagement.

I applaud Dr. Alterio for a clear presentation of Dr. Reilly's contributions to the biosocial core of occupational therapy knowledge. I was one of Dr. Reilly's graduate students at the University of Southern California and, along with my colleagues in the program, contributed to the knowledge base in the evolving occupational behavior frame of reference (as Reilly termed it at the time). We studied literature predominantly drawn from the behavioral sciences on the broad areas of play, work, intrinsic motivation, rules, interests, time, occupational choice, and occupational role behavior through the life cycle. Clinically, we did occupational and play histories to identify skills and achievements in good order and deficit areas needing intervention. We constructed play and productive work environments in our practice settings as we strove to develop skills of the individuals we treated. Dr. Reilly would say: "Skills are to OTs what pills are to MDs."

Dr. Alterio presents thorough descriptions of prominent practice models and describes how they can be integrated into an occupation-based model. The chapters overall are informative, clear, easy-to-follow, and well referenced. Of particular interest are his fascinating accounts of the key events, individuals, and cultural forces that influenced the formation and growth of occupational therapy practice and education. This text also includes thoughtful discussions of contemporary issues related to public health, occupational science, ethics, and the globalization of the occupational therapy profession.

The individuals with whom we work cover the entire age span and have significant insults to their minds and bodies because of illness, injury, deviations in development, and/or poor living conditions. They share the commonality that engagement in meaningful and purposeful daily occupations is significantly impaired. Individuals in our caseload, whether in hospitals, rehabilitation centers, schools, or community facilities, present many challenges. It is critical and very practical to adopt a sound conceptual model to guide the complexities of occupational therapy practice.

Dr. Alterio offers students, instructors, and practitioners a lively discussion of relevant topics enhanced by his unique perspective based on 30 years of practice and 15 years as an educator. This excellent text deserves wide readership encompassing both educational and professional circles.

Linda Florey, PhD, OTR/L, FAOTA
Former Chief, Rehabilitation Services
Resnick Neuropsychiatric Hospital at UCLA
Los Angeles, California

Preface

In occupational therapy, theory is important because it tells us what to expect. Theory is a framework for practitioners because it provides a structure for perceiving and solving problems. Theory is a framework for educators who conduct research to validate practice approaches and pass on knowledge to students who will be future practitioners. Theory is a framework for the public because it represents the profession's social contract and establishes guidelines for what people can expect from its practitioners.

Our profession sometimes lacks agreement about how and when various practice theories are applied. That may be partially due to the wide range of practice areas in which occupational therapists work. The demands of a pediatric intensive care nursery are very different from a clubhouse for adolescents with substance abuse problems or a home environment where someone is trying to arrange care for a parent with dementia. Occupational therapists work in all these settings and many others, but without theory, practice devolves into pragmatic and context-specific methods that can lack central coherence.

I wrote this book with the aim of addressing this concern. In more than 30 years of practice, I have worked in many different settings and have seen many approaches to providing occupational therapy services. Over the course of my career, there have been numerous changes to health care systems, and occupational therapy became a worldwide profession. I've witnessed the profession's struggle to emerge into a Third Paradigm and to integrate its scientific advances while maintaining a focus on the core value of occupation.

When I was a student, my mentor, Kent Tigges, told me that every person who needed my help would be a test for the profession's central premise as articulated in occupational behavior theory. I was gifted with that educational heritage, and in many settings and in providing intervention to thousands of people, I learned repeatedly that when we understand the complexity of people's needs and the impact of broad systems on occupations, our services can be coherently directed, effective for problem solving, and, most importantly, meaningful to those we serve.

This text builds on that simple formula: that we should be *not only* concerned with our basic science, *but also* constantly mindful of how that science impacts the person, family, community, and society related to occupation. This integration constitutes the science and art of occupational therapy practice.

The book is primarily intended to be used as a college-level textbook, particularly for courses dedicated to theory and the development of the occupational therapy profession. It is also designed to be helpful for practicing clinicians who are interested in reviewing theory to support an integration of practice approaches.

This text is divided into three parts. Section 1 provides important historical information about the profession's philosophy and core values. This material serves as a foundation for understanding paradigm changes that occurred over time and how the field has evolved into its current state as a care-providing profession. Section 2 includes discussion of important approaches and models and how they can be integrated in clinical practice. Section 3 includes an exploration of emerging practice and new practice models, including a call to critically reflect on how these ideas apply in everyday practice settings.

Each chapter includes learning objectives, key terms, and review questions to help the reader organize study and reinforce understanding of the material. Individual, small-group, and full-class learning activities are provided to encourage research and critical-thinking skills. Selected chapters include case studies and case study questions to facilitate making the connection between theory and practice. All chapters include references listing relevant supporting literature.

Occupational therapists frequently find themselves in a position of needing to explain the nature and scope of their services. My hope is that this book can also contribute to clarifying our role by providing a concise overview of what practitioners, educators, and the public can expect from occupational therapy.

Christopher J. Alterio

Acknowledgments

Writing a book is a team-oriented occupation, and I am grateful to so many people who made this project possible. Thank you to Michael Nobel, for seeing merit in my original idea and for introducing me to the wonderful team of professionals at Wolters Kluwer. Thank you also to Kerry McShane and Amy Millholen, whose encouragement and support helped keep this project on target.

I want to express extra special thanks to Tanya Martin, my development editor, whose guidance and feedback was instrumental in shaping this text. You never know how much you need a development editor until you work with someone like Tanya. I can't thank her enough.

I am very grateful for all the content reviewers who provided excellent feedback and suggestions for improving the book. I appreciate the efforts of so many people who helped with photographs: my dear friend Dee Berline, Nicole Schmidt from ABC Therapeutics, who helped hold the fort and provide assistance with photos, and Clare Byrne from Imprint Hope for her photos and inspiration. Thanks also to all my other family members, friends, and patients, who made important photographic contributions. Thank you so much!

I am very grateful for the contributions of my Keuka College occupational therapy graduate students. Emily Good led the team with obtaining permissions for photographs and illustrations, and I need to credit Brittany Mendel and Ashlee Lytle for helping to unearth historical documents and photos long forgotten in library archives. These students and many others provided important support for researching the history chapters.

I want to thank the occupational therapy faculty at Keuka who thought it would be interesting to add the extra challenge of Division Chair during an accreditation year to my responsibilities as I was writing—but their unending support and friendship made it all possible. I am privileged to work with this faculty, and they provided a lot of feedback, encouragement, and laughs along the way. Of course, the keystone of my Keuka family support is Sandy Teague, whose everyday administrative wizardry allowed me to multitask and actually have an appearance of competence. I could not have written this book without all this support.

There are so many intangible acknowledgments that I want to make. I am thankful to my first occupational therapy theory instructor, Phillip Shannon, who carried the intellectual heritage of Mary Reilly into his own classroom and passed it along to his students. I am forever grateful to my mentor and friend, Kent Tigges, who showed me how to take the concepts of occupational behavior and put them directly into practice. Another mentor and friend, Peter Talty, provided me with many professional opportunities that supported my ability to take on this project.

I am thankful to all my friends and colleagues at the National Board for Certification in Occupational Therapy (NBCOT). Over many years of volunteer work, I have been mentored and supported by so many knowledgeable colleagues and leaders—too numerous to count—but their cumulative impact on my professional development is beyond measure. In particular, I am very thankful to Linda Florey, another of Mary Reilly's students, who was so gracious with her willingness to write a Foreword. I met Linda during my work with NBCOT. She has been a professional and leadership inspiration, mentor, and a good friend. It is an honor to have her contribute to this effort and represent the intellectual heritage that serves as the foundation of this book.

I also want to thank the many occupational therapy colleagues who have been so willing to engage in conversation and debate in person and online and who have helped me with my critical thinking and professional growth. All these experiences are written between the lines of this book.

Finally, I want to thank my family and, in particular, my wife Caroline. Her unending love and willingness to endure the obsession required to produce a textbook made this possible. She is my foundation, and everything she does makes it possible for me to do everything that I do.

Reviewers

Alma R. Abdel-Moty, Dr.OT, MS, OTR/L
Clinical Associate Professor
Academic Fieldwork Coordinator
Nicole Wertheim College of Nursing and
Health Sciences
Florida International University
Miami, Florida

Karen Brady, D.Ed, OTR/L
Assistant Professor
Department of Occupational Therapy
The University of Scranton
Scranton, Pennsylvania

Elizabeth Cara, PhD, OTR/L, MFCC
Professor Emerita
Department of Occupational Therapy
College of Applied Sciences and Arts
San Jose State University
San Jose, California

Paula Carey, OTD
Associate Professor of Occupational Therapy
Utica College
Utica, New York

Gregory Chown, OTD, OTR/L, BHSc(OT),
BA, CPAM, CKTP
Associate Professor
Occupational Therapy Program
Alvernia University
Reading, Pennsylvania

Cassady Hoff, MS
Occupational Therapy Assistant Program
Director
School of Health Science
Casper College
Casper, Wyoming

Veronica T. Rowe, CBIST, MS(R), PhD,
OTR/L, FNAP
Assistant Professor
Department of Occupational Therapy
University of Central Arkansas
Conway, Arkansas

Linda S. Russ, PhD, OTR
Assistant Clinical Professor
Occupational Therapy Department
D'Youville College
Buffalo, New York

Aricka Schweitzer, MSOT, OTRL, C/NDT
Assistant Professor of Occupational Therapy
Saginaw Valley State University
University Center, Michigan

Contents

Development and Growth of the Occupational Therapy Profession

1   Key Concepts and Core Values

Occupation is as necessary to life as food and drink. . ... Every human being should have both physical and mental occupation. . ... Sick minds, sick bodies, sick souls, may be healed through occupation.

—William Rush Dunton[1]
Reconstruction Therapy

Chapter Outline

Learning Objectives

1. Define the terms *occupation* and *occupational therapy (OT)*.
2. Provide examples of common practice settings for OT.
3. Differentiate between a theory, a paradigm, and a model and explain how each relates to OT practice.
4. List and define the seven core values of the OT profession that are part of the Occupational Therapy Code of Ethics of the American Occupational Therapy Association (AOTA).
5. List and define the six key principles of professional conduct that are part of the Occupational Therapy Code of Ethics.
6. Explain how professional ethics guide the choices a therapist makes in practice.

Key Terms

autonomy
beneficence
ethics
fidelity
justice
model
models of practice
nonmaleficence
occupation
occupational therapy
paradigm
practice setting
theory
veracity

Overview

Occupational therapy (OT) is a caring profession that has a core belief that occupation is central to health and happiness. Over time, there have been changes in definitions, practice settings, and ethical codes that impact the practice of OT. These changes also influence the development of theory that is used to guide practice decisions. In this introductory chapter, two brief case studies are used to provide beginning examples of how some of these different factors intersect with the way that OT professionals gather information, solve problem, and create intervention plans. It is important to understand how practice settings, theories, and ethics are all used to organize the provision of OT services.

What Is Occupational Therapy?

The word *occupation* is commonly used in our society to refer to a person's job or profession. In the practice of occupational therapy (OT), the term has a broader, more holistic meaning. **Occupation** refers to the activities of daily living, including self-care, education, work, play, leisure, social participation, rest, and sleep.

In the past, occupation has been described in ways that range from simple to complex. The American Occupational Therapy Association (AOTA)[2] defined occupation as the ordinary and familiar things that people do every day. In contrast, Pierce[3] stated that occupation consisted of an individual's personally constructed, nonrepeatable subjective experience that is perceived in personally unique ways. She differentiates occupations from activities by stating that activity is a culturally defined and general class of human action.

Occupational therapists' clinical decision making is guided by the belief that occupation is central to human life and happiness and that problems with occupational engagement contribute to ill-health and poor adaptation. Occupation is a requisite for a good life. These are fundamental beliefs that have been consistently articulated since Meyer[4] wrote the first philosophy of OT.

Occupational therapy is the health care profession that focuses on helping people of all ages do the things they want and need to do in daily life. Occupational therapists use occupations to promote health and wellness, to remediate or restore function, to maintain health, and to prevent disease and injury.[5] OT professionals provide services to assist a wide range of individuals in living the best life possible in spite of illness, injury, or disability. Occupational therapists work in many different practice settings and help people participate not only in essential daily activities but also in those that they find meaningful.

There have been serial changes to the definition of OT just over the past two decades. The AOTA Practice Framework[6] defined the profession as follows:

> Occupational therapists and occupational therapy assistants focus on assisting people to engage in daily life activities that they find meaningful and purposeful. Occupational therapy's domain stems from the profession's interest in human beings' ability to engage in everyday life activities.

Just a few years later, in the AOTA Practice Framework, 2nd edition,[7] the definition was changed:

> Within this diverse profession, the defining contribution of occupational therapy is the application of core values, knowledge, and skills to assist clients (people, organizations, and populations) to engage in everyday activities or occupations that they want and need to do in a manner that supports health and participation.

In the AOTA Practice Framework, 3rd edition,[8] the definition of OT was changed again:

> Occupational therapy is defined as the therapeutic use of everyday life activities (occupations) with individuals or groups for the purpose of enhancing or enabling participation in roles, habits, and routines in home, school, workplace, community, and other settings. Additionally, "the clients of occupational therapy are typically classified as persons (including those involved in care of a client), groups (collectives of individuals, eg, families, workers, students, communities), and populations (collectives of groups of individuals living in a similar locale—eg, city, state, or country—or sharing the same or like characteristics or concerns). Services are provided directly to clients using a collaborative approach or indirectly on behalf of clients through advocacy or consultation processes."

Wholesale changes to the definition of OT had a wide-ranging impact on theory and practice in the past and continue to influence contemporary study and practice.

Practice Settings

A **practice setting** refers to the environment in which OT services are delivered. The role of the therapist will vary according to the environment and the patients/clients served. Common practice settings include the following:

- Medical and nursing facilities (eg, inpatient, outpatient, rehabilitation, assisted living, long-term care)
- Schools and other educational facilities
- Community locations (eg, private practice offices, senior centers, supported living communities)
- In-home care
- Virtual environments (eg, telerehabilitation, synchronous or asynchronous online spaces)

Each environment has its own set of mandated rules that influence and direct action within the setting. The different contexts that occupational therapists work within sometimes make therapy look different in different places and can influence the tools and methods the therapist might use (Figure 1-1).

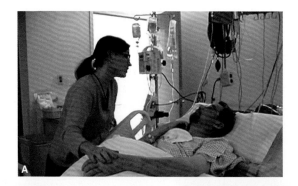

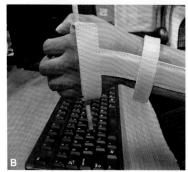
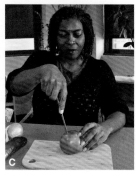

Figure 1-1   Occupational therapists work with individuals in a variety of practice settings. A, Therapist in a hospital intensive care unit, assessing a person who had a stroke. B, Assistive devices may be used to help students perform school-related tasks. C, Therapists work in home settings to help individuals successfully perform daily tasks such as food preparation. (Reprinted with permission from Boyt Schell BA, Gillen G, Scaffa ME, Cohn ES. *Willard and Spackman's Occupational Therapy*. 12th ed. Philadelphia, PA: Lippincott Williams & Wilkins/Wolters Kluwer; 2013.)

Theory As the Basis for Practice

A **theory** is a set of ideas intended to explain a phenomenon or serve as a set of principles on which some type of practice is based. A **paradigm** is a broad perspective or a shared set of ideas across a particular group or profession. A paradigm serves several functions: it reflects the purpose of a profession, describes the nature and scope of its practice, describes the content of its educational curricula, and guides its research interests.[9] Over the past century, OT practice has been shaped by a number of fundamental theories and paradigms, which will be discussed in later chapters.

A **model** is a device used to represent or stand for an object or idea through the use of a physical or symbolic form. Models are useful in suggesting ideas or methodologies, providing alternatives, and analyzing situations and conditions.[10]

Models of practice are important for explaining both why and how a discipline organizes its knowledge and directs action. Conceptual practice models in OT have a theoretical base, along with a research and evidence base, to guide the use of various tools and methods. The varied practice models used by occupational therapists allow for a diverse range of interventions that can be used to achieve each individual's unique treatment goals.

The Occupational Therapy Code of Ethics

Ethics are defined as the moral principles that govern a person's behavior. The OT profession is guided by core values and ethical principles outlined in the AOTA Code of Ethics. The core values are intended to guide practitioners toward ethical behavior in professional and volunteer roles, and the principles present standards of professional conduct that apply to AOTA members.

The AOTA core values are as follows:

- *Altruism*: acting on the basis of concern for the welfare of others
- *Equality*: treating all people equally, without prejudice or bias
- *Freedom*: using the right of personal choice in a responsible manner
- *Justice*: ensuring fair treatment across all individuals served, populations, and communities
- *Dignity*: respecting the patient/client at all times
- *Truth*: communicating clearly, accurately, and honestly
- *Prudence*: exercising effective reasoning skills and sound judgment

The six key principles embodied in the AOTA Code of Ethics are **beneficence**, **nonmaleficence**, **autonomy**, **justice**, **veracity**, and **fidelity** (Figure 1-2). The values and ethics of the OT professional are demonstrated every day as therapists interact with patients/clients and their family members, other health care professionals, and community members.

Ethics in Action

The following two vignettes provide examples of how ethical principles direct the therapist's choices and actions.

AOTA Code of Ethics

Beneficence
- Occupational therapy personnel shall demonstrate a concern for the well-being and safety of the recipients of their services.

Nonmaleficence
- Occupational therapy personnel shall refrain from actions that cause harm.

Autonomy
- Occupational therapy personnel shall respect the right of the individual to self-determination, privacy, confidentiality, and consent.

Justice
- Occupational therapy personnel shall promote fairness and objectivity in the provision of occupational therapy services.

Veracity
- Occupational therapy personnel shall provide comprehensive, accurate, and objective information when representing the profession.

Fidelity
- Occupational therapy personnel shall treat clients, colleagues, and other professionals with respect, fairness, discretion, and integrity.

Figure 1-2   Summary of the key principles and standards of conduct of the Occupational Therapy Code of Ethics. AOTA, American Occupational Therapy Association. (Source: The American Occupational Therapy Association. Occupational therapy code of ethics (2015). *Am J Occup Ther.* 2015;69(suppl 3):6913410030. doi:10.5014/ajot.2015.696S03.)

CASE 1-1 *Billy*

Billy is 6 years old. He is sitting quietly in his first-grade classroom and sees a friendly looking woman approach.

"Hi Billy!" the woman says. "My name is Miss Keary, and I'm an occupational therapist. Your teacher said it would be okay if I helped you with your letters today."

Before this visit, the occupational therapist had reviewed Billy's Individualized Education Program and noticed that he was scheduled to receive special education support, speech therapy, and the OT that she was asked to provide.

As Miss Keary sat down, Billy remembered that he had an "OT teacher" who came to his preschool program, and he feels comfortable with this new person.

"How are you doing with your letters?" Miss Keary asked. "I was looking at some of your papers, and I think you're doing a really great job with trying to keep them all on the line!"

"Sometimes my letters get all wiggly," Billy replied. "My OT teacher always used to sing a song to me and it helped me remember to start my letters on the top."

Miss Keary watched Billy as he struggled to control the pencil in his hand. His letters were poorly formed and not always legible. These observations were consistent with the reports she had read earlier. She also noticed that the worksheet he was using had very small spaces where he was supposed to write.

"I think that singing that song is a great idea!" she told him. "Maybe we can also try using a different pencil and different paper, too. I think this is going to make learning these letters a lot of fun!"

Analysis

Miss Keary, the occupational therapist, demonstrated commitment to several key ethical principles. First, she approached Billy with a notable concern for his well-being and ability to learn in school. This aligns with the principle of beneficence (taking action to help others). The therapist also demonstrated a concern for Billy's autonomy in wanting to help him develop skills so he could be independent with his learning activities. She also demonstrated the principle of fidelity by treating Billy with respect and by engaging him within the expected scope of practice of the OT profession.

In this example, therapy is being provided in the school setting, under a U.S. educational mandate that all children, including those with disabilities, have a right to a free and appropriate public education. There are corresponding rules and regulations that dictate the boundaries of the therapy services that can occur within the educational context. The therapist plans to use several approaches chosen for the purpose of helping Billy with the important occupation of writing.

1. Schools must adhere to privacy laws that protect all students. The right to confidentiality in a school setting would be represented by which ethical principle?
2. Sometimes, families and school districts disagree on what services should be provided to a child. Which ethical principle should be considered when determining if a student's right to an education has been respected?
3. What ethical principles should guide the occupational therapist's recommendations in a meeting during which services are being determined by the educational team?

CASE 1-2   *Sue*

Sue walked gingerly into the outpatient OT department and followed the therapist to a private room where the evaluation would take place.

"What bad luck I've had lately!" Sue exclaimed. She reported that she was involved in a motor vehicle crash 2 days ago but had previously scheduled the appointment for other reasons. She initially went to the doctor because of pain in her hands and lower back. The physician thought that sitting at a computer for many hours a day, as she did in her job as a paralegal, might be causing the problems. "Now I'm sore all over my body."

"Does your doctor know that you were in a car accident?" the therapist asked. He looked at the referral that requested an ergonomic assessment and a home program to address her pain.

"I think the emergency room sent him the x-rays. They said nothing was broken but that I'd probably be sore for a few days. I'm supposed to follow up with him, but now I don't have transportation. I had to ask a friend to bring me here today."

The therapist told Sue that he could do some basic assessment and send a report to the doctor right away. He continued, "Then we can ask for an updated referral in case he wants us to do anything different based on the ER report and our assessment. Before your next appointment with me, it will be good for you to follow up with your doctor."

The therapist completed the evaluation and included assessments of Sue's range of motion, strength, posture, motor coordination, and pain levels. He also interviewed her about her work and asked if she could take some pictures of her workstation to send to him.

"Thank you so much," Sue exclaimed. "I really think this is going to help. Now the only thing I need to figure out is if I need to pay a copay or whether this should be billed to the auto insurance because of the accident."

"Insurance issues can be complicated," he replied. "Let's talk to the billing people, and we'll also need some input from your doctor about that. I know we can get it straightened out for you."

Analysis

The occupational therapist demonstrated commitment to several ethical principles. He was concerned about Sue's well-being (beneficence), and he also took specific actions so that he would avoid causing harm (nonmaleficence). He did this by ensuring that Sue's doctor knew about the accident and by sending information to the doctor's office so an updated referral could be given. He demonstrated the principle of veracity by carefully documenting his assessment findings and taking steps to determine which payer should be billed for his services.

In this case, therapy services are being provided in a medical setting (an outpatient therapy clinic), and some form of private insurance will be billed. The doctor sent Sue to this facility for an ergonomic assessment, and she has an expectation of coordinated care between the therapist and the doctor.

1. Would it ever be ethically or legally acceptable for the occupational therapist to leave billing determinations exclusively to the facility billing department? Why or why not?
2. Would it ever be ethically or legally acceptable to refuse to treat a patient if he or she arrives at the facility with a different set of problems than those listed on the referral? How would a therapist decide what to do in this situation?
3. If the therapist knows that a patient does not have transportation and might not be able to follow up with his or her doctor, what is the most ethical course of action?

Summary

- In the field of OT, *occupation* refers to the activities of daily living, including self-care, education, work, play, leisure, social participation, rest, and sleep. Occupation is central to human life and happiness.

- OT focuses on helping people of all ages do the things they want and need to do in daily life. Therapists use occupations to promote health and wellness, to remediate or restore function, to maintain health, and to prevent disease and injury.

- OT may be provided in a wide range of practice settings, including within medical and educational facilities, in private clinics and other community locations, and in private homes. OT practice is influenced by the practice setting (environment) in which services are provided.

- A theory is a set of ideas intended to explain a phenomenon or serve as a set of principles on which a practice is based. A paradigm is a broad perspective shared across a particular group or profession. A model is a representation of a structure, an idea, or a set of actions.

- Conceptual practice models in OT have a theoretical base, along with a research and evidence base, to guide the use of various tools and methods.

- The seven core values of the AOTA Occupational Therapy Code of Ethics are altruism, equality, freedom, justice, dignity, truth, and prudence.

- The six key principles of professional conduct that are part of the AOTA Occupational Therapy Code of Ethics are beneficence, nonmaleficence, autonomy, justice, veracity, and fidelity.

- The values and ethics of the OT profession guide therapists as they interact with patients/clients, colleagues, and community members.

Reflect and Apply

Individual activity

Reflect on volunteer or personal experiences where you have seen people who were ill or disabled. Consider the following questions and note your responses.

1. How did you and other people interact with the person?
2. What ethical principles may have guided any of those interactions?
3. In what setting did these interactions occur?
4. Was the person unable to participate in some occupations because of his or her condition or location?

5. What type of assistance may have been needed to help that person engage in occupations?
6. Did you see an occupational therapist interact with the person? If so, describe the therapist's interactions.

Small group discussion

After noting your individual responses, form a small group and discuss your observations with other group members.

Review Questions

1. A physician has asked for a progress note on a patient. The occupational therapist asks the patient to sign a release form to grant permission for a picture to be taken of the hand for documentation purposes. The use of the release form shows that the therapist is acting on the basis of the ethical principle of

   a. veracity.
   b. justice.
   c. autonomy.
   d. beneficence.

2. An occupational therapist is asked by a supervisor to change the date on some treatment notes, and the therapist knows that this is not legal. The therapist is concerned about the ethical principle of

   a. veracity.
   b. justice.
   c. autonomy.
   d. beneficence.

3. An occupational therapist sees a patient with a diagnosis with which the therapist has little experience. The therapist informs the client that she will be transferred to another therapist who has more experience with this medical condition. The therapist who was originally assigned to this client is acting on the basis of the ethical principle of

   a. veracity.
   b. justice.
   c. autonomy.
   d. beneficence.

4. An occupational therapist is interested in providing consultation services via computer to patients in another state (telerehabilitation), but must apply for licensing and learn

all applicable rules that govern this method of practice. The therapist is concerned with the ethical principle of

a. veracity.
b. justice.
c. autonomy.
d. beneficence.

5. An occupational therapist is offered a part-time position providing weekend home visits for an early intervention agency. The therapist currently works for another agency that provides the same services and is concerned about conflict of interest if she accepts the part-time job. Her concerns are related to the ethical principle of

a. veracity.
b. fidelity.
c. autonomy.
d. nonmaleficence.

6. An occupational therapist is found guilty of a driving-while-impaired infraction and is instructed by the court to enroll in outpatient counseling and report their offense to the appropriate regulatory and licensing agencies. In complying with this order, the therapist is respecting the ethical principle of

a. veracity.
b. fidelity.
c. autonomy.
d. nonmaleficence.

7. An occupational therapist has been working in an elementary school and is interested in a new job in an assisted living facility. This new opportunity represents a primary change in

a. ethics.
b. model of practice.
c. practice setting.
d. values.

8. An occupational therapist working with children who have learning difficulties hears about a new treatment approach in a social media networking group. The new approach is different from what is currently used at his place of employment. The therapist should describe this to the supervisor as an opportunity to learn about a new

a. code of ethics.
b. model of practice.
c. practice setting.
d. set of values.

References

1. Dunton WR. *Reconstruction Therapy*. Philadelphia, PA: W.B. Saunders Company; 1919.
2. The American Occupational Therapy Association. Position paper: occupation. *Am J Occup Ther*. 1995;49:1015-1018. doi:10.5014/ajot.49.10.1015.
3. Pierce D. Untangling occupation and activity. *Am J Occup Ther*. 2001;55:138-146. doi:10.5014/ajot.55.2.138.
4. Meyer A. The philosophy of occupational therapy. *Arch Occup Ther*. 1922;1:1-10.
5. The American Occupational Therapy Association. The philosophical base of occupational therapy. *Am J Occup Ther*. 2011;65(suppl):S65. doi:10.5014/ajot.2011.65S65.
6. American Occupational Therapy Association. Occupational Therapy Practice Framework: Domain & Process. *Am J Occup Ther*. 2002;56(6):609-639.
7. American Occupational Therapy Association. Occupational Therapy Practice Framework: Domain & Process, 2nd Edition. *Am J Occup Ther*. 2008;62(6):625-683.
8. The American Occupational Therapy Association. Occupational therapy practice framework: domain and process (3rd edition). *Am J Occup Ther*. 2014;68(supp 1):S1-S48. doi:10.5014/ajot.2014.682006.
9. Shannon P. The derailment of occupational therapy. *Am J Occup Ther*. 1977;31(4):229-234.
10. Reed KL. *Models of Practice in Occupational Therapy*. Baltimore, MD: Williams and Wilkins; 1984.

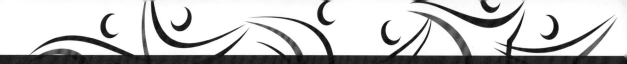

2 The Historical Context of Occupational Therapy

It is the purpose of history to elucidate connections in hope that we can learn from our rich past and feel more related to it.

—Kathleen Barker Schwartz[1]
Eleanor Clarke Slagle Lecture

Chapter Outline

Learning Objectives

1. Explain the value of understanding the history of occupational therapy.
2. Describe how early occupation workers were influenced by the Moral Treatment Movement, Transcendentalism, and the Arts and Crafts Movement.
3. Describe key aspects of the Gilded Age that played a role in the social movements of the time.
4. List the professional disciplines that contributed to early occupation work.
5. Describe the role of George Barton and other founders in the establishment of the National Society for the Promotion of Occupational Therapy.
6. Explain how World War I affected the development of the occupational therapy profession.
7. Identify some early methods used by occupational therapists as treatment.
8. State the original definition and philosophy of occupational therapy.
9. Differentiate between *rest cure* and *work cure*.
10. Explain what is meant by the *paradigm of occupation*.
11. State the purpose of practice standards and educational standards for the emerging occupational therapy profession.

Key Terms

educational standards
founders
moral treatment
paradigm of occupation
philosophy
practice standards
reconstruction aides
rest cure
settlement house
work cure

Overview

Occupational therapists have an important covenant with their history. When we commit ourselves to studying history, we can develop a deep understanding that allows us to reflect upon the meaning of our profession. We can benefit from studying broad social and cultural movements because they help us understand the development of people in social and cultural contexts over time. Knowledge of key movements provides a perspective on how they influenced the founding and growth of the occupational therapy profession.

Founders are individuals who create a new enterprise. Learning about the people involved in establishing the occupational therapy profession can be just as illuminating as studying the historical context of their times.

In this chapter, we will discuss important historical events and contexts that contributed to the profession's founding. We'll also focus on people who were doing "occupation work" before the profession officially existed, as well as those who were formally involved in its founding. Understanding the broad range of opinions, methods, and motivations of the founders allows us to understand not only how the profession was established but also the basis for the theory that serves us in practice today.

The Gilded Age

The late 19th century in American history is known as the Gilded Age. The term was coined by Mark Twain and Charles Dudley Warner in their novel, *The Gilded Age: A Tale of Today*, originally published in 1873, which depicted the rise of the modern industrial economy and the underlying greed and corruption behind many of the fortunes made at this time.

During this period, industrialization was transforming the nature of people's work from small independent enterprises into industrial corporations located in major urban areas (Figure 2-1). A new wave of European immigration was occurring, bringing with it a steady supply of labor and resulting in unprecedented population growth. Electricity and telecommunications were introduced into cities, and railroads were built that connected distant areas of the country. All of these events contributed to the dramatic societal change of this era.

Massive wealth was accumulated during the early stages of industrialization by a select few, accompanied by a very deep level of poverty among the masses. The poor lived in

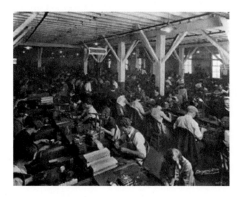

Figure 2-1   Factory workers in New York City, 1894.

unsanitary conditions, medical treatments were crude or unavailable, and chronic illnesses such as tuberculosis presented major social problems.

The movements that occurred during this time arose in response to extreme social upheaval. Most were attempts to improve the living conditions of the population and were based on the principles of charity, philanthropy, and Christian ethics. Noting the severe struggles of working people, Pope Leo XIII issued the *Rerum Novarum*, an important encyclical on the rights and duties of capital and labor that was critical of the excesses of capitalism and concerned with the rights of working people. The lack of social supports at the time led other religious organizations to also take steps to address social problems. The Emmanuel Movement (discussed later in this chapter) is an example of such efforts. Lay efforts such as the Arts and Crafts Movement were aimed at ameliorating the negative impacts of industrialization and rapid social change. The occupational therapy profession was forged in the crucible of this age.

Moral Treatment Movement

The philosophy of **moral treatment** arose as part of the broad 18th-century European Enlightenment. Prior to this time, mentally ill individuals were often physically restrained and abused. Several notable reformers took action to improve the state of care of people in asylums.

French physician Philippe Pinel (1745-1826) suggested that environmental changes could affect an individual's psychology and thereby change behavior. He was director of asylums in Paris and known as a pioneer in the humane treatment of the mentally ill. In England, Quaker philanthropist William Tuke (1732-1822) employed similar methods at the York Retreat in England, where patients were housed in a pleasant environment, fed properly, and could engage in normal daily tasks. In the United States, these ideas were put into action by Philadelphia physician Benjamin Rush (1746-1813), a signer of the Declaration of Independence.[2]

By today's standards, the efforts of these reformers could be considered crude or primitive, but their visionary beliefs contributed to the emergence of the occupational therapy profession. They were convinced that mental health conditions could be medically treated. Their methods were based on compassion and respect and on providing opportunities for normal participation in occupations as part of treatment programs.

American Transcendentalism

To *transcend* means to go beyond the limits of something. American Transcendentalism is a philosophy that arose in the 1820s and 1830s, mainly in Boston and New England, which emphasized the value of the spiritual and transcendental over the material. A core belief was in the independence and self-reliance of individuals, which was consistent with the thinking of several occupational therapy founders discussed later in this chapter.

Transcendentalists believed in the inherent goodness of people and nature and were committed to creating a uniquely American literature and philosophy. In Boston, Ralph Waldo Emerson, Henry David Thoreau, Amos Bronson Alcott, Margaret Fuller, and others were key members of this group.[3] A principle tenet emphasized individual freedom and harmony with nature. In 1837, Emerson wrote the now-famous lines:

> *We will walk on our own feet; we will work with our own hands; we will speak our own minds... A nation of men will for the first time exist, because each believes himself inspired by the Divine Soul which also inspires all men.*

Arts and Crafts Movement

The Arts and Crafts Movement emerged in England, Europe, and North America as a response against industrialization and its impact on the lives of working people and their environments. The movement protested the decline in aesthetic and quality standards that resulted from the shift to mass-produced home goods and worked to support individual craftsmanship in the decorative and fine arts. William Morris (1834-1896), an architect, artist, and textile designer, was at the forefront of this movement in England. This oft-repeated Morris quote captures the spirit of the movement: "Have nothing in your houses that you do not know to be useful, or believe to be beautiful."

George Barton, a Bostonian and one of the founders of the occupational therapy profession, studied architecture. He was apprenticed to William Morris and played a role in bringing the ideals of the Arts and Crafts Movement to the United States.[4]

The Origins of Occupational Therapy

The beginnings of the occupational therapy profession occurred in context with broader social changes and changing approaches to the treatment of mental and physical illness in the United States. The founders of the profession were challenged to create a definition and philosophy describing their work and then move on to developing educational and practice standards.

Many of the early proponents of using "occupation" as a form of treatment arrived at their methods through their respective fields. Professionals who participated in "occupation work" came from diverse backgrounds and included physicians, nurses, teachers, social workers, counselors, ministers, architects, and artisans. Table 2-1 lists some prominent members of this original group.

Table 2-1

People and Professions Influential in the Development of Occupational Therapy

NAME	PROFESSION	NOTABLE ACCOMPLISHMENTS
William Rush Dunton	Medicine	Physician and original OT founder Pioneer in promoting occupational therapy methods
Herbert Hall	Medicine	Physician and founder of Devereaux Mansion Pioneer in promoting occupational therapy methods
Adolph Meyer	Medicine	Physician and author of the philosophy of occupational therapy
Thomas Kirkbride	Medicine	Physician and moral treatment pioneer Believed that architecture and environment could promote health
Susan Tracy	Nursing	Pioneer in nursing education on the use of occupations Invited to NSPOT founding meeting but could not attend.
Reba Cameron	Nursing	Reconstruction aide Pioneer in nursing practice on the use of occupations
William James	Psychology/Counseling	Known as the "father of American psychology" Applied Transcendentalism to psychological thought
Elwood Worcester	Psychology/Counseling	Leader of the Emmanuel Church of Boston and founder of the Emmanuel Movement
Samuel McComb	Psychology/Counseling	Associate rector of the Emmanuel Church and prolific writer on its efforts
Eleanor Clarke Slagle	Social Work	Original OT founder Pioneer in organizing and developing occupational therapy into a professional discipline
Julia Lathrop	Social Work	Social reformer and Hull House collaborator with Jane Addams
Wilfred Grenfell	Social Work	British physician and medical missionary Introduced economic self-sufficiency for the indigenous populations of Labrador and Newfoundland, Canada
Susan Cox Johnson	Arts and Crafts Education	Original OT founder and artisan educator Advocated for crafts as a therapeutic method
Jessie Luther	Arts and Crafts Education	Artisan and pioneering occupation worker who worked with Grenfell in Labrador and Newfoundland
Ora Ruggles	Arts and Crafts Education	Reconstruction aide who wrote a novel that popularized early occupation work
George Barton	Architecture	Architect and original OT founder Founder of Consolation House
Thomas Kidner	Architecture	Canadian architect and original OT founder International liaison for occupational therapy

Abbreviations: NSPOT, National Society for the Promotion of Occupational Therapy; OT, occupational therapy.

Early occupation workers did not always agree on common definitions, scope of practice, or methods. They modified and clarified practice based on their experiences and relied on leadership from key members among their ranks and on the medical leadership that would help establish legitimacy for their developing efforts.

George Barton and Consolation House

George Edward Barton (1871-1923) was a member of the social elite in Boston who traveled widely and was tutored by famous designers and intellectuals. When he returned to the United States, he became a member of elite social clubs such as the Tavern Club in Boston, where he continued to cultivate contacts with other wealthy people.[5]

George Barton had access to education and many professional and social opportunities. But his life of privilege did not spare him from disease and disability. In 1901, he contracted tuberculosis and moved to Denver to benefit from fresh air and exercise as part of his recovery.

Barton's early architectural work included designing the South Bay Union, part of the South End House project, a **settlement house** project intended to assist Boston's poor, immigrant population (see Box 2-1 for more on settlement houses). While in Colorado, he continued his interest in socially driven architecture by developing the Myron Stratton Home in Colorado Springs, a residence for the poor, including displaced children, orphans, and senior citizens.[4]

In 1912, Barton suffered another health setback when he lost part of a foot to frostbite while on a survey assignment. He relocated to Clifton Springs, New York, to receive care at a well-known sanitarium. This is where Barton met Dr Elwood Worcester, an Episcopal priest and pastor of the Emmanuel Church in Boston,[6] who also held a PhD in psychology. Worcester was founder of the Emmanuel Movement, which originated in 1906 as a psychological approach to healing conditions known at the time as *neurasthenia*. These "nervous" conditions included depression, anxiety, other mental and emotional problems, fatigue, and addictions. Worcester and fellow priest Samuel McComb established a free clinic at the church and used a combination of spiritual counseling, relaxation techniques, and suggestion to treat those who sought their help. Barton was one of Worcester's patients.[7]

In 1917, Isabel Newton, Barton's wife, wrote, "The Rev. Elwood Worcester, of Emmanuel Church, Boston, convinced him that perhaps living was not worth the effort for himself, it would be worthwhile to get well for the sake of the 'other fellow.' With this inspiration, Barton set out to discover what could be done for others suffering from illness and disability."

Consolation House

Consolation House opened in March 1914, and marked the beginning of Barton's efforts that ultimately led to the incorporation of the Consolation House Convalescent Club on April 1, 1922. Barton's earlier experience as a member of elite social clubs served as the basis for his creation of a new kind of club. The purpose of the Convalescent Club was to provide a place where disabled individuals could rehabilitate themselves and develop skills for economic

BOX
2-1

Settlement Houses

The Settlement House Movement originated in London in the late 1880s as a way to provide education and social services for impoverished workers. Settlement houses were to serve as a mechanism for supporting people through social and cultural integration. These endeavors were funded by the charitable efforts of reform-minded people who wanted to improve living conditions and social outcomes.

The movement carried over to the United States, and settlement houses were established in New York, Boston, Chicago, and other cities to improve the lives of workers and to assist immigrants in transitioning into the labor force and American life. George Barton was well known for his contributions in this area and with his partner won the Shattuck prize for the development of artisan homes.[25] He also designed buildings as part of the South End Movement in Boston.[4] Other occupational therapy founders were also linked with this movement, most notably Eleanor Clarke Slagle with her work in Chicago.[9] ∎

self-sufficiency. Every article or product made by a disabled person was to be stamped with the image of a phoenix, the official emblem of Consolation House (Figure 2-2). Barton chose the phoenix to represent his belief that something new could be born out of his loss.

Each product was also to be stamped *Beauty for Ashes* so buyers would know that "this article was made by a sick man who is doing his very best to support himself."[8] The motto *Beauty for Ashes* reflects Barton's spiritual conversion. It is based on a Biblical passage (Isaiah 61:3) asserting that people who have suffered loss can be comforted, consoled, and find happiness again.

Consolation House was aptly named. Barton came to believe that he had a mission, and fulfilling that mission was an expression of hope for his own recovery as well as the recovery of others in similar situations. As part of his work with Consolation House, Barton communicated with others who were using occupation as a therapeutic tool. This group of innovators ultimately came together to formally establish the basis for occupational therapy as a profession.

Other Key Founders

The degree of collaboration and influence among early occupation workers is remarkable, given the relatively primitive state of communication technology in the early 1900s.

Psychiatrist *William Rush Dunton* (1868–1966) is another important figure in occupational therapy history and played a significant role in implementing the moral treatment philosophy at the hospital where he worked.[9] Dunton began corresponding with Barton in 1914. Through their collaboration, Barton was introduced to the work of other key professionals:

- *Thomas Kidner* (1866-1932) was an English vocational education and rehabilitation expert who became Vocational Secretary of the Canadian Military Hospitals Commission.

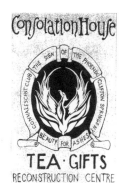

Figure 2-2   Consolation House emblem showcasing the phoenix, a beautiful bird originating in Egyptian and Greek mythology that symbolizes rebirth and triumph over death and difficulty. (Reprinted with permission from Clifton Springs Historical Society.)

- *Adolf Meyer* (1866-1950) was a psychiatrist who integrated everyday life skills into mental health treatment. He was the founding director of the Henry Phipps Psychiatric Clinic at Johns Hopkins Hospital.
- *Eleanor Clarke Slagle* (1870-1942) was a social worker with experience in the care of the disabled. Meyer hired her as director of occupational therapy at Johns Hopkins, where she served for 2 years before becoming superintendent of occupational therapy for Illinois state hospitals.
- *Susan Johnson* (1876-1932) was a teacher and nurse who specialized in using crafts as a therapeutic tool.
- *Susan Tracy* (1864-1928) was a nurse who established the occupational therapy department at Chicago's Presbyterian Hospital.
- *Herbert James Hall* (1870-1923) was a physician who established a private facility in Massachusetts for the treatment of "nervous disorders."

Defining a New Profession

Correspondence between Dunton and Barton resulted in their choosing the name the National Society for the Promotion of Occupational Therapy (NSPOT) for their professional association. Slagle initially disagreed with the use of the term *therapy* and expressed a desire to subdivide the topic into educational, economic, and therapeutic areas. Barton insisted upon retaining *therapy* because he felt it was important to emphasize the health-giving aspect (vs the commercial aspect), and Dunton agreed with Barton's stance. The first meeting of the NSPOT convened on March 15, 1917 at Consolation House (Figure 2-3).

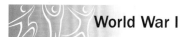 ## World War I

On April 6, 1917, just weeks after the NSPOT organizational meeting, the United States declared war on Germany. The NSPOT founding members were determined to investigate ways that the new Society could participate in the war effort. Barton called upon Thomas

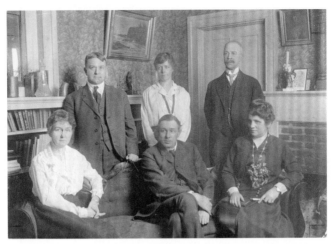

Figure 2-3   Founders of occupational therapy at the first meeting of the National Society for the Promotion of Occupational Therapy, March 1917 at Consolation House. Front (left to right): Susan Cox Johnson, George Barton, Eleanor Clarke Slagle. Back (left to right): William Rush Dunton, Isabel Gladwin Newton, Thomas Kidner. (Photo from author's private collection.)

Kidner to leverage his US and Canadian military contacts to help organize programs that would benefit soldiers.

In June 1917, Barton reached out to Frank Gilbreth, a US Army engineer who served on a panel making recommendations for reeducation work for wounded soldiers. Barton also reached out to international contacts he was attempting to involve in the process.

Reconstruction Aides

In World War I, **reconstruction aides** were civilian women who provided treatment in the form of physical and occupational therapy (Figure 2-4) to assist in the rehabilitation of servicemen who had been wounded and/or were suffering from *battle neurosis*, the condition we know today as posttraumatic stress disorder. There were not enough occupation workers to meet the wartime demand. While some were nurses, others were recruited to the cause and accepted based only on their experience as artisans or teachers.

There was little standardization in regard to prior experience and training of the reconstruction aides. As a result, the activities that service members were engaged in varied widely, often dependent on the skill and preferences of the individual aide. A very basic level of instruction was reviewed by the fledgling NSPOT. In spite of this lack of standardization, reconstruction aides' efforts were widely praised by medical directors, and occupational therapy activities were publicized because of the positive message about reengagement and participation that they exemplified.[10]

After the war, many reconstruction aides returned to their prior work as artisans and teachers, while others continued with formal occupational therapy training. The inherent

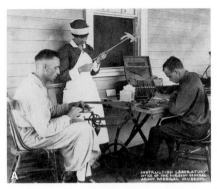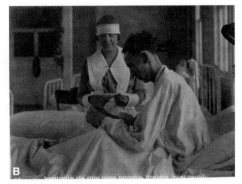

Figure 2-4   A, Wounded World War I soldiers being taught scroll work by reconstruction aide at Walter Reed Hospital, Washington, DC (Source: Reeve Photograph Collection, National Museum of Health and Medicine). B, Reconstruction aides providing bedside instruction at Fitzsimons General Hospital, Aurora, CO (Source: National Library of Medicine).

challenges of role delineation between occupational and physical therapists, the need for educational standards, and debates related to the value of diversional versus therapeutic orientations are professional issues that emerged from this early form of occupational therapy.[10]

Establishing Standards for a New Profession

The meeting at Clifton Springs was an important event in the early development of occupational therapy, but naming a professional organization and convening a small number of motivated disciples is very different than the work required to advance a new profession. Early practitioners were influenced by the social, cultural, and economic forces of their time (Figure 2-5). They were challenged by the fact that the medical system they functioned within was also in a state of early development. There were inconsistencies in the ways that illness and disease were understood and inconsistencies in medical practice. Modern diagnostic and treatment methods were in their infancy.

Among the OT founders, there were differences of opinion on the nature of the developing profession. Adolph Meyer published his seminal statement on the philosophy of occupational therapy in 1922, but at the time there were many divergent opinions and methods being used and no unifying beliefs or system of practice.

Influence of the Rest Cure and Work Cure

The **rest cure** (extended bed rest) was first promoted by Philadelphia physician Silas Weir Mitchell in the 1870s as a treatment for nervous conditions. Patients were cared for totally, with nurses feeding them milk and stimulating their muscles with primitive

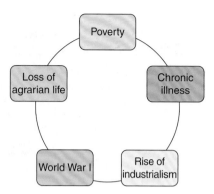

Figure 2-5   Converging social and economic forces in the United States at the time of the founding of the occupational therapy profession.

electrotherapy devices to prevent muscle atrophy. This treatment was mainly prescribed for women.

Some ideas related to the rest cure carried over into early occupational therapy. Patients were provided nonstrenuous activity for diversional purposes, to keep their mind free from worry about their condition while they spent long periods of time in medical confinement.

In contrast, the **work cure** was promoted by early Emmanuel Movement doctors as part of their overall treatment method. It is based on the philosophy of engaging the patient in useful activities and developing skills as part of recovery (**Figure 2-6**). In 1908, Richard Cabot,[11] a Massachusetts physician and pioneer of medical social work, wrote a treatise on the work cure and suggested that therapeutic work should be immersive, pragmatic, and socializing. "Cabot's theory of how this would be therapeutic was a mixture of Transcendentalism, Jamesian habit training, social psychology, and cognitive restructuring."[12] This same methodology was being considered and applied by Adolph Meyer and Eleanor Clarke Slagle at the Henry Phipps Psychiatric Clinic at Johns Hopkins Hospital in Baltimore.

These Emmanuelist methods inspired Dr Herbert Hall[13] who advocated occupation and activity to engage patients and to stimulate their physical and psychological recovery. He and New England artist Jessie Luther refined these methods at Devereaux Mansion and later inspired the same approach at the Sanitarium at Clifton Springs.[14]

The Paradigm of Occupation

Many people engaging in early occupation work had inconsistent levels of training, and there was a corresponding variation in the skills that these individuals brought to their work.[10] Early occupation workers practiced their trade in different parts of the country and approached their work from a variety of perspectives, but all shared a common belief in the use of occupation as a treatment modality. This focus became known as the **paradigm of occupation**.

In the early stages of any endeavor, dissemination of ideas and agreement about concepts is necessary for consensus building and consistency. **Figure 2-7** highlights significant

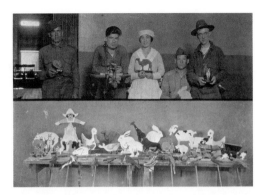

Figure 2-6   Toy making in a psychiatric hospital. This activity was widely used as part of the rehabilitation of wounded World War I soldiers (Source: Reeve Photograph Collection, National Museum of Health and Medicine).

events in the early history of OT. A professional **philosophy** is a statement that outlines the theoretical basis for a profession. The new occupational therapy profession relied heavily on the leadership of medical doctors to develop a defining philosophy that would be respected in the broader medical community.

In 1921, Dr Adolph Meyer[15] offered his philosophy of occupational therapy, which was read at the Fifth Annual NSPOT Meeting. Meyer's philosophy focused on the value of time and work as enduring concepts that organized human life. He identified the action-orientation of human beings and suggested that balanced living was achieved through participation in work, play, rest, and sleep. He believed that human satisfaction arose from autonomy and opportunity and that occupational therapists should strive to provide these for their patients. This philosophy was the undisputed basis for American occupational therapy for many years.

The NSPOT agreed on a definition for the profession supplied by Dr Harry A. Pattison[16]; he stated that occupational therapy was "any activity, mental or physical, definitely prescribed and guided for the distinct purpose of contributing to, and hastening, recovery from disease or injury."

Practice Standards

Despite the publication of a philosophy and definition, not all early occupation workers would have been aware of these statements, and some may not have agreed with them. Many years passed during which the definition and practice of occupational therapy was open for interpretation.

Practice standards are defined as a set of guidelines and criteria for providing care. The occupational therapy definition went through additional changes and refinement in accordance with varying local interpretations, but "a new formal definition of occupational therapy did not appear again for nearly 50 years."[17]

The work required to put occupational therapy into action was monumental. Eleanor Clarke Slagle documented her methodology for introducing occupational therapy programs into hospital systems in New York State. Her efforts introduced consistent practice standards

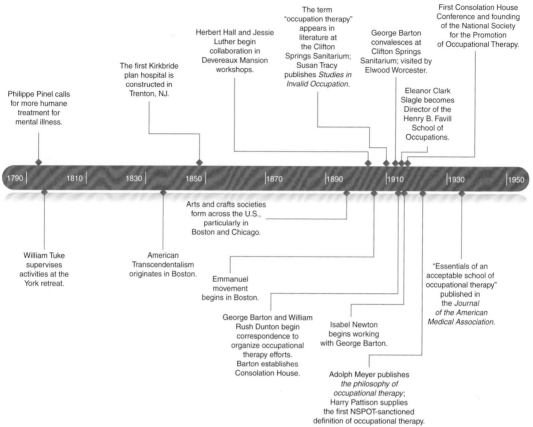

Figure 2-7   Significant events in the early history of occupational therapy. NSPOT, National Society for the Promotion of Occupational Therapy.

in terms of requiring a doctor's prescription for therapy and focusing on habit training. Her methods also incorporated a level of flexibility in regard to how each department or facility would implement their programs. She stated, "Our first step was toward a unified program of occupational therapy; but one which would, at the same time, allow of wide individual freedom to the superintendents of the various hospitals. In other words, we felt that our duty to the work called for an attitude of advisory helpfulness towards those directly responsible for the care and treatment of the patients, rather than an attitude of 'direction.'"[18]

It was very difficult for Slagle to implement this standardization because of the diverse ways in which occupational therapy had been historically practiced. Slagle acknowledged that occupational work historically developed through a humanitarian phase, an economic phase, and a therapeutic phase[19] (Figure 2-8). Specific goals were associated with each phase. The perception that occupations should be diversional, recreational, and of economic benefit persisted for many years (even among some leaders in the field), despite Slagle's standardization efforts.

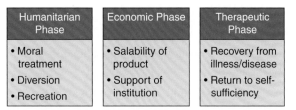

Figure 2-8   Historical phases of occupation work and the primary goals of each phase.

Educational Standards

Educational standards are criteria that state what students should be taught as part of a specific academic or training program. Slagle is credited with creating the first formalized OT training program at the Henry B. Favill School of Occupations. The program included 5 months of training in social service, administration, kinesiology, gymnastics, and craft work.[20] Later training programs promoted by Brackett[21] and Hall[22] modeled the Boston School of Occupational Therapy and also included coursework in medical topics.

After many years of debate, the American Medical Association (AMA) was invited to oversee the accreditation process for occupational therapy educational programs. The 1935 Essentials[23] introduced significantly greater rigor into occupational therapy training programs, including a minimum of 100 hours of training in medical topics, social sciences, therapeutic media, and a robust experiential component. AMA oversight also marked the beginnings of a relationship with medicine that significantly influenced the ongoing development of the profession.[24]

Summary

- Studying the history of occupational therapy helps students and practitioners develop a more complete understanding of the purpose and meaning of the profession.

- Early occupation workers were influenced by the compassionate ideals of the Moral Treatment Movement, by the belief in individual freedom and self-reliance associated with Transcendentalism, and the respect for individual craftsmanship rooted in the Arts and Crafts Movement.

- The modern industrialism and greed of the Gilded Age led to a backlash of social movements that emphasized the rights of the worker and harmony with nature.

- Early occupation work was influenced by professionals in medicine, nursing, social work, psychology/counseling, teaching, architecture, and arts and crafts.

- George Barton and other key OT founders established the NSPOT to define the profession and advance its mission and goals.

- The reconstruction aides of World War I provided physical and occupational therapy to wounded soldiers and veterans in the United States and overseas.

- Early OT methods included engaging patients in useful activities associated with work and recreation.

- The earliest formal definition of occupational therapy was "any activity, mental or physical, definitely prescribed and guided for the distinct purpose of contributing to, and hastening, recovery from disease or injury."

- The rest cure incorporated extended bedrest. In contrast, the work cure involved productive tasks, exposure to the outdoors, and physical exercise.

- The *paradigm of occupation* refers to the use of occupation as a treatment modality for illness and disability.

- Practice standards provide guidelines for how the tasks of a particular profession are to be performed; in health care, these are standards for providing care.

- Educational standards establish requirements for academic and training programs.

Reflect and Apply

Individual activities

1. Conduct online research into the biographies of historical occupational therapy figures. What information can you learn to help you better understand the work they did to establish the profession?
2. Compare and contrast the occupational therapy and physical therapy professions. If the two professions had been combined, how do you think health care would be different today?

Small group discussion

1. How does the current debate about the level of training needed for occupational therapy practitioners compare with the debates on this topic at the profession's inception? What social forces influence this issue? Should OTs be trained at a doctoral level? Should OT assistants be trained at a baccalaureate level?
2. How does the early debate on relevant occupations relate to modern-day practice? Is there a place for arts and crafts in modern occupational therapy?
3. Early OTs had difficulty developing consensus around standards of practice. Do modern information-sharing networks solve or create problems with creating consensus and standards for occupational therapy? Consider this question as it relates to regional, national, and international information sharing.

Read and discuss

Makerspaces, also called *hackerspaces*, are collaborative work spaces in public or private facilities where people build or create with materials, learn how to share resources, and work together to make something of interest to them. They are found in libraries, schools, and community centers, and people are invited to come to these locations to work on individual or shared projects.

In the early 20th century, occupational therapy makerspaces were created in sanitariums as part of treatment for convalescing tuberculosis patients. Contemporary occupational therapists are becoming interested in makerspaces once again because of the concept of a constructed milieu where people come together to develop skills.

1. What drives the makerspace movement today?

2. Is it appropriate for makerspaces to be located in libraries, schools, and even in home improvement stores? Why or why not?

3. What is the role of occupational therapy in contemporary makerspaces?

Review Questions

1. Occupational therapy's original roots were *not* influenced by

   a. social Darwinism.
   b. moral treatment.
   c. arts and crafts philosophy.
   d. Transcendentalism.

2. Which of the following is most associated with moral treatment?

   a. Society has a moral right to institutionalize people who are mentally ill.
   b. Society has a moral obligation to help those with mental illness return to a normal life pattern.
   c. Society has no moral obligation to normalize disorganized behavior.
   d. Society is most concerned with "survival of the fittest" as a moral response to disorganization.

3. Transcendentalism was primarily focused on

   a. human freedom and an individual's harmony with nature.
   b. the promotion of a welfare state.
   c. a new focus on meditative practices.
   d. establishing international norms for social justice.

4. Name the Boston architect who studied with William Morris and later became a founder of the occupational therapy profession.

   a. Richard Clipston Sturgis
   b. Ralph Adams Cram
   c. George Edward Barton
   d. William Rush Dunton

5. The purpose of the Arts and Crafts Movement was to emphasize the

   a. importance of governmental subsidy of the arts.
   b. need to promote fair wages and working conditions for artisans.
   c. dangers of social utopias being considered by European philosophers.
   d. value of a return to aesthetics in design in response to industrialization.

6. Which of the following terms was used by Mark Twain to describe a time period that was full of opportunity but also driven by underlying corporate greed?

   a. The melting pot
   b. The Gilded Age
   c. Industrialism
   d. The Social Gospel

7. Name the Emmanuelist practitioner and minister who "treated" George Barton and set him on a path to play a key role in the development of the occupational therapy profession.

   a. Adolph Meyer
   b. William Morris
   c. Elwood Worcester
   d. Herbert Hall

8. Name the Canadian architect whose presence at the Consolation House meeting was expected to help attract international interest in the new occupational therapy profession.

   a. Thomas Kidner
   b. James Lougheed
   c. Marcus Paterson
   d. Jules Amar

9. Name the doctor who was not invited to the Consolation House meeting but nonetheless went on to be president of NSPOT and make many contributions to the occupational therapy profession.

   a. Adolph Meyer
   b. Susan Tracy

   c. Susan Cox Johnson

   d. Herbert Hall

10. Name the doctor who practiced at the prestigious Sheppard-Pratt Hospital and was responsible for initiating the correspondence that led to the organization of NSPOT.

   a. Adolph Meyer

   b. Jules Amar

   c. William Rush Dunton

   d. Herbert Hall

11. Name the OT founder who worked in Chicago and was responsible for starting the Henry B. Favill School of Occupations.

   a. Eleanor Clarke Slagle

   b. Susan Cox Johnson

   c. Isabel Gladwin Newton

   d. Susan Tracy

12. Name the doctor who published the seminal statement on the philosophy of occupational therapy.

   a. William Rush Dunton

   b. Adolph Meyer

   c. Herbert Hall

   d. Jules Amar

13. Which form of occupation was used to help patients cope with long periods of bed restriction while under orders for a "rest cure?"

   a. Recreational

   b. Diversional

   c. Restorative

   d. Economic

14. In addition to the use of suggestion and spiritual counseling, the Emmanuelists promoted the idea of

   a. work cure.

   b. rest cure.

   c. moral treatment.

   d. habit training.

15. The occupation workers who treated injured soldiers during World War I were called

   a. doughboys.

   b. occupational nurses.

    c. reconstruction aides.

    d. rehabilitation teachers.

16. The earliest official definition of occupational therapy was

    a. the use of occupation designed to promote balanced living.

    b. any activity, mental or physical, prescribed and guided for the distinct purpose of contributing to, and hastening, recovery from disease or injury.

    c. the therapeutic application of arts and crafts to promote health.

    d. diversional, economic, and rehabilitative use of occupation during periods of illness or disease to encourage balance and return to ordinary living.

17. Which OT founder was responsible for promoting both practice and educational standards for the developing profession?

    a. Susan Cox Johnson

    b. George Edward Barton

    c. William Rush Dunton

    d. Eleanor Clarke Slagle

References

1. Schwartz KB. Reclaiming our heritage: connecting the Founding Vision to the Centennial Vision [Eleanor Clarke Slagle lecture]. *Am J Occup Ther*. 2009;63:681-690. doi:10.5014/ajot.63.6.681.
2. Goodwin CJ. *A History of Modern Psychology*. 5th ed. Hoboken, NJ: John Wiley & Sons; 2015:340-345.
3. Gura PF. *American Transcendentalism: A History*. New York, NY: Hill & Wang; 2007:XII.
4. Meister M. *Arts and Crafts Architecture: History and Heritage in New England*. Hanover, Germany: University Press of New England; 2014.
5. de Lancey B. George Edward Barton: Undaunted cripple's courage aided others. *The Geneva Times*. May 9, 1958:2.
6. Barton GE. *Teaching the Sick: A Manual of Occupational Therapy and Re-education*. Philadelphia, PA: W.B. Saunders & Co; 1919.
7. Barton IG. Consolation House, fifty years ago. *Am J Occup Ther*. 1968;22:340-345.
8. Helping convalescents to help themselves. *Trained Nurse Hosp Rev*. 1922;68(5):432-433.
9. Quiroga V. *Occupational Therapy: The First 30 Years*. Bethesda, MD: AOTA Press; 1995.
10. Low JF. The reconstruction aides. *Am J Occup Ther*. 1992;46(1):38-43.
11. Cabot R. Work cure. *Psychotherapy*. 1908;3(1):28.
12. Ernst W. *Work, Psychiatry, and Society c. 1750-2010*. Manchester, England: Manchester University Press; 2016.
13. Rompkey R. *Jessie Luther at the Grenfell Mission*. Montreal, QC, Canada: McGill-Queen's University Press; 2001:xxix.
14. Husted MI. The industrial department at Clifton Springs. *Clifton Med Bull*. 1913;1(1):27-28.
15. Meyer A. The philosophy of occupational therapy. *Arch Occup Ther*. 1921;1(1):1-10.
16. Pattison HA. The trend of occupational therapy for the tuberculous. *Arch Occup Ther Rehabil*. 1922;1:19-24.
17. Reed KL, Sanderson SN. *Concepts of Occupational Therapy*. 4th ed. Philadelphia, PA: Lippincott Williams & Wilkins; 1999:5.

18. Slagle EC. A year's development of occupational therapy in New York State Hospitals. *Mod Hosp.* 1924;22(1):98-104.

19. Scullin V. *Occupational Therapy: Manual of Reference for Personnel.* Albany, NY: New York State Department of Mental Hygiene; 1956:9-12.

20. Loomis B. The Henry B. Favill School of Occupations and Eleanor Clarke Slagle. *Am J Occup Ther.* 1992;46(1):34-37.

21. Brackett EG. Scope of occupational therapy and requirements for the training of occupational aides. *Arch Occup Ther.* 1922;1(3):179-186.

22. Hall HJ. Occupational therapy in 1921. *Mod Hosp.* 1922;18:61-63.

23. American Medical Association. Essentials of an acceptable school of occupational therapy. *J Am Med Assoc.* 1935;104:1631-1633.

24. Colman W. Structuring education: development of the first educational standards in occupational therapy, 1917-1930. *Am J Occup Ther.* 1992;46:653-660.

25. Barton IG. *Talk Given Before the Western New York Occupational Therapy Association at the Clifton Springs Sanitarium.* Ontario, NY: Clifton Springs Sanitarium; 1947.

3 Twentieth-Century Paradigm Shifts

Our profession emerged from a common belief held by a small group of people. This common belief is the hypothesis upon which our profession was founded. It was, and indeed still is, one of the truly great and even magnificent hypotheses of medicine today . . .. That man, through the use of his hands as they are energized by mind and will, can influence the state of his own health.

—Mary Reilly[1]
Eleanor Clark Slagle Lecture

Chapter Outline

Learning Objectives

1. Define habit training and explain how it applied to occupational therapy in the 1920s.
2. Explain what is meant by *reductionism* in regard to science and the practice of occupational therapy.

3. Explain why the occupational therapy profession had an interest in aligning with medicine in the mid-20th century.
4. Identify early medical leaders of the occupational therapy profession.
5. Identify occupational therapists who developed and promoted reductionistic models of practice in the 20th century.
6. Describe the paradigm crisis caused by the profession's embracing medical models of practice.
7. State how Mary Reilly and her students played significant roles in refocusing the profession toward occupation-based models of practice.
8. List the principles of occupational behavior that led to the development of the model of human occupation.

Key Terms

habit training
medical model
model of human occupation
occupational behavior model
paradigm shift
paradigm crisis
reductionism

Overview

The occupational therapy profession was founded on the ideals that occupation is important and that it adds both meaning and purpose to life. Occupations were used as an intervention strategy as well as an outcome objective. In the first half of the 20th century, external pressure from the medical profession, combined with occupational therapists' desire to gain acceptance, led to a gradual shift from the original focus on occupation to an emphasis on medical models of practice. Although these medical models were important and helpful in expanding the scientific basis of the profession, they did not clarify or support occupational therapy's unique contribution and purpose as a health profession.

In 1961, Mary Reilly initiated a critical inquiry into the relative value of the occupational therapy profession through her Eleanor Clarke Slagle lecture. Her work and that of her students challenged the profession to reexamine its historical roots and led to the development of more occupation-based models of practice that would become the profession's focus for many years. This chapter traces the profession's evolution from its initial focus on occupation, to a more medical and mechanistic emphasis, to the late 20th-century shift back to occupation, supported by the scientific and technological advances of this era.

The 1920s and Habit Training

Recall from Chapter 2 that psychiatrist Adolf Meyer was an important early influence on the emerging OT profession. He was named Director of the Henry Phipps Psychiatric Clinic at John Hopkins based on his expertise in psychobiology, the combined nature of physical and mental concerns.

Meyer's[2] philosophy of occupational therapy can be summarized as follows:

> The whole of human organization has its shape in a kind of rhythm, always kept up to a standard at which it can meet rest as well as wholesome strain without upset. There are many other rhythms which we must be attuned to: the larger rhythms of night and day, of sleep and waking hours, of hunger and its gratification, and finally the big four—work and play and rest and sleep, which our organism must be able to balance even under difficulty. The only way to attain balance in all this is actual doing, actual practice, a program of wholesome living as the basis of wholesome feeling and thinking and fancy and interests. . ... Our role consists in giving opportunities rather than prescriptions. There must be opportunities to work, opportunities to do and to plan and create, and to learn to use material.

Meyer recruited Eleanor Clarke Slagle to help implement his ideas about **habit training** and achieving a healthy balance of work, play, rest, and sleep. In habit training, daily activities were closely planned, scheduled, and supervised until patients could assume and maintain those habits on their own.[3]

Slagle worked to implement Meyer's philosophy and successfully spread this concept through training courses and the organization of various institutional and hospital departments. Their combined efforts were critical to the development of the new occupational therapy profession.

The Second Paradigm: Reductionism

Reductionism is defined as a philosophic approach in which complex ideas are understood by breaking them down into smaller parts. During the 1930s and following World War II, significant advances in science and technology were changing the way that physicians understood and treated illness and disease. The entire field of medicine experienced enormous change because of the introduction of imaging technology, research that led to new ways of understanding disease processes, and advances in pharmaceuticals and surgical techniques. From the 1930s through the 1950s, medicine and other health-related professions adopted reductionistic approaches based on enhanced and more sophisticated scientific knowledge. These science-based methods are known as the **medical model**.

The concept of occupation is very complex, and there was strong pressure for occupational therapists to more clearly define and articulate the science behind their efforts. Early occupational therapy leaders turned to the medical profession for patronage and direction; this relationship with medicine had a notable impact on the developing OT profession. Physicians and others in medically related disciplines provided important leadership, and the greatest impact they had was on the development of professional standards, increasing professionalism, and promoting a scientific basis for research.

This wide-scale shift from a focus on occupation to an emphasis on addressing specific physical and mental impairments and disabilities is known as a **paradigm shift**. Basic assumptions about the role and function of the occupational therapist changed when practice was based on the medical model. Kielhofner[4] retrospectively referred to this new focus as the *mechanistic paradigm*, in which occupational therapists adopted the values and perspectives of medicine.

Leaders From the Medical Profession

Dr C. Floyd Haviland (Figure 3-1) was an important physician-leader for the occupational therapy profession. Recruited by Eleanor Clarke Slagle[5] he was instrumental in organizing and developing occupational therapy departments during his tenure as member and Chairman of the New York State Hospital Commission. He served as American Occupational Therapy Association (AOTA) president from 1928 to 1929. After his untimely death on January 1, 1930, he was succeeded for a brief interim by Thomas Kidner and then by Dr Joseph Doane (1931-1939; Figure 3-2) and Everett Elwood (1939-1947; Figure 3-3).

Figure 3-1   C. Floyd Haviland, MD (Courtesy of the Archive of the American Occupational Therapy Association, Inc.)

The creation of a national registry of qualified practitioners and establishing standards for educational programs were debated for several years before both were implemented in 1935. AOTA board members had divergent opinions on what educational standards should be.[6] At that time, there were many different pathways into the profession. The matter was ultimately settled under Dr Doane's presidency.

Doane's leadership reflected a kind but paternalistic view of occupational therapists, who were subservient within the medical hierarchy. He encouraged his charges to "be alert, be tactful, be hard working—these three, but the greatest of these is tact."[7] He was concerned about the lack of science in occupational therapy and encouraged therapists to abandon the use of arts and crafts.[8] Kidner and Doane collaborated on efforts to have the American Medical Association take responsibility for accrediting occupational therapy training programs.[6]

Figure 3-2   Joseph Doane, MD (Courtesy of the Archive of the American Occupational Therapy Association, Inc.)

With professional leadership provided primarily by male physicians, occupational therapists struggled between wanting autonomy and still finding "credibility and security" under medical patronage.[9] This dynamic was also influenced by the slow pace of social change in regard to gender roles at that time. Occupational therapy leaders through the 1940s and 1950s often adopted research pathways that paralleled the interests of their physician patrons.

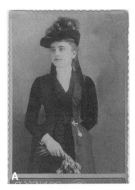 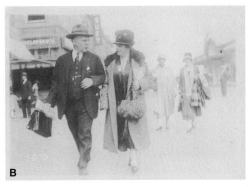

Figure 3-3   A, Young Eleanor Clarke Slagle. B, Everett Elwood and Eleanor Slagle at the American Occupational Therapy Association conference in Atlantic City, NJ, 1937. (Courtesy of Fenimore Art Museum Research Library.)

Reductionistic Methods Used for Physical Disabilities

In the mid-20th century, several theoreticians with expertise in physical therapy developed treatment protocols that crossed over into the occupational therapy arena. Their work exemplified the growing focus on reductionistic science as both rehabilitation professions adopted aspects of their theoretical frameworks.

Berta Bobath (1907-1991) was a physical therapist who collaborated with her husband, a psychiatrist/neurophysiologist, to develop new treatment techniques for stroke patients and children with cerebral palsy. She published extensively in physical therapy and occupational therapy journals. Bobath's methods became known as the Bobath concept/approach or neurodevelopmental treatment and were used with both pediatric and adult populations.[10]

Figure 3-4   Margaret S. Rood (Courtesy of the Archive of the American Occupational Therapy Association, Inc.)

Margaret S. Rood (1909-1984; Figure 3-4) was trained as both an occupational therapist and physical therapist and emphasized a research-based approach to treatment. She was instrumental in developing treatment approaches for children and adults with motor impairments due to central nervous system disorders. In particular, she focused on a developmental model of reflex and motor control and techniques to facilitate or inhibit abnormal muscle tone and reflexes that were limiting normal movement.[11]

Signe Brunnstrom (1898-1988) was a Swedish-American physical therapist and educator who adopted the findings of Twitchell[12] and formulated a developmental progression of recovery following central nervous system injury.[13] Her methods were widely adopted by occupational therapists working with adults who had cerebral vascular accidents.

Figure 3-5   A. Jean Ayres (Courtesy of the Archive of the American Occupational Therapy Association, Inc.)

A. Jean Ayres (1920-1988; Figure 3-5), an occupational therapist, clinical psychologist, and educator, developed a theory of sensory integration[14] and was at the forefront of researching and developing treatment methods for individuals with neurologic impairments in sensory integration.

Other occupational therapists[15,16] also serve as exemplars of how occupational therapists built on scientific knowledge to develop a more precise understanding of how the human body functions in normal development and in the presence of illness, disability, and disease. All of these 20th-century theorists/practitioners made important contributions to the scientific advancement of the rehabilitation professions, and many of their methods are still in use today.

Reductionistic Methods Used for Mental Health Treatment

Dr Fern Cramer-Azima and her husband Dr Hassan Azima provided important contributions to the application of psychodynamic treatment ideas into occupational therapy.[17] Dr Cramer-Azima developed the Azima Battery,[18] a projective test that has been broadly used by occupational therapists to assess mood, drives, and object relations with the intent of aligning treatment with approaches favored by psychiatry.

Gail Fidler and her husband Dr Jay Fidler also provided important seminal contributions to the role of occupational therapy using a psychodynamic approach.[19] Their focus on activity analysis and communication during the therapeutic process[20] was an important basis for occupational therapy models for many years.

Gail Fidler influenced many other prominent occupational therapists, notably *Anne Cronin Mosey*, who made important contributions to organizing occupational therapy knowledge into frames of reference for mental health interventions. Her work in this area went on to have broad influence on occupational therapy philosophy and theory development.

These leaders, along with many others, worked to legitimize occupational therapy's role in mental health treatment. They accomplished this objective by focusing on the accepted psychodynamic theories that were in use at the time. They also made contributions to the occupational therapy field that were influential beyond their initial theoretical purposes.

Derailment of the Profession?

Some occupational therapists look at the period from the 1950s through the 1970s and believe that occupational therapy "lost sight of the paradigmatic values and beliefs of its founders."[21] Specifically, Shannon stated that the profession aligned itself with the medical model, failed to speak out against medicine's failure to meet the needs of the chronically disabled through the rehabilitation movement, and that there was a devaluing of the principles that originated with the Arts and Crafts Movement. He labeled this process a "derailment" of the profession.

The medical leadership during this time created a contextual shift in the "normal science" of occupational therapy. This normal science[22] is typically composed of efforts directed toward clarifying, proving, and disproving ideas that were expressed in the original articulation of the paradigm. So, normal science for the first paradigm of occupation would have been directed toward testing initial assumptions and concepts when the profession was initially formed. That process never really happened, and instead, occupational therapists began to focus on the scientific objectives of their new patron/leaders in medicine. Shannon was concerned that there was a disconnection between occupational therapy's initial purpose and the way it was being practiced under medical leadership.

Influential occupational therapy leaders who hoped to refocus the profession on its original values were critical of reductionistic approaches (see Box 3-1). However, reductionistic methodologies were important in the development of the profession, and many OT professionals made contributions to patient care by focusing their efforts on small component aspects of human functioning. Adopting biomechanical models, traditional motor control models, and psychodynamic models provided a point of commonality between the growing occupational therapy profession and the scientific values of other disciplines. The challenge with these reductionistic approaches was that they did not always provide clarity and distinction for occupational therapy as a unique profession.

Resolution of the Paradigm Crisis

A **paradigm crisis** occurs when questions emerge about the shared values and beliefs of a scientific community or professional group.[22]

In its first paradigm (1917-1930s), the occupational therapy profession identified itself as a field that appreciated the importance of occupation in human life, addressed problems of occupational disengagement, and used occupation as a therapeutic measure. In its second paradigm (1940s-1970s), the profession changed its focus to regarding human performance as intact biomedical functions and operated at the level of remediating those dysfunctional factors that were impeding function. These two conflicting perspectives represented the first true paradigm crisis in the occupational therapy profession.

Mary Reilly (1916-2012; Figure 3-6), an occupational therapist and educator, addressed the paradigm crisis in her 1961 Eleanor Clarke Slagle lectureship. Reilly believed that occupational therapy required a third paradigm, in which the profession reidentified itself as primarily concerned with human occupation and directed toward understanding the human need for work and productivity.

For Reilly, the central question was whether or not occupational therapy was "a sufficiently vital and unique service for medicine to support and society to reward." This inquiry into the value of occupational therapy is still relevant for therapists today. Reilly believed that the gap between disability or dysfunction and the nature of occupational therapy interventions at that time was a barrier because of an inadequate understanding of people's need for productivity and how active engagement contributed to health and wellness. She did not believe that occupational therapy had adequately explained its methods and, as a result, the profession was drifting into accepting the medical system's models.

Figure 3-6   Mary Reilly (Courtesy of the Archive of the American Occupational Therapy Association, Inc.)

Reilly believed that the human need for action was universal and that "human nature does not thrive in idleness." She believed that the unique service of occupational therapy was in addressing the "need to master [the] environment—to alter and improve it." She stated that "the mind and will of man are occupied through central nervous system action, and man can and should be involved consciously in problem solving and creative activity." This premise has been criticized by some occupational therapists as being too Western in its orientation.[23]

BOX   3-1

BOX   3-1

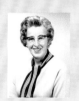

Wilma West (Courtesy
of the Archive
of the American
Occupational Therapy
Association, Inc.)

Beatrice Wade
(Courtesy of
the Archive of
the American
Occupational Therapy
Association, Inc.)

Steps Toward Independence

Wilma West, MA, OTR, FAOTA, was AOTA executive director from 1947 to 1951 and founder and President of the American Occupational Therapy Foundation from 1972 to 1982. During the 75th anniversary year, West[36] reflected on "Ten Milestone Issues in AOTA History." In this article, she expressed her belief that "loosening control by physical medicine" was the most important milestone issue in AOTA history. Although the close relationship with medicine was important for occupational therapy's development, a time came for the profession to reject medical patronage and avoid exclusive medical control.

West stated that the effective argument made by *Beatrice Wade*, director of the occupational therapy program at the University of Illinois, Chicago, convinced AOTA's Education Committee and Board of Management to issue a policy statement of independence in 1950. This resulted in the occupational therapy profession gaining control of the registry of approved therapists and of establishing and maintaining educational and professional standards (previously responsibilities of the American Medical Association).

This policy statement was a critical turning point for the profession. It loosened the singular control of the growing field of physiatric medicine, established occupational therapy as a profession with broad relationships with other medical specialties, and promoted the beginning of professional autonomy. ■

AOTA, American Occupational Therapy Association.

According to Reilly, occupational therapy's problem was not reductionistic models of psychiatry and rehabilitation, but that those ideas were not properly incorporated into the profession's unique area of contribution—human engagement and productivity. She stated,

> There is a long, perilous and complex ladder to be scaled between neuro-muscular efficiency and work satisfaction. The ontogenetic reconstitution of motor behavior is a tedious process and must be done step by step . . . if any of these steps are missing, they must be refashioned and the whole pattern reshaped accordingly. The proof of the occupational therapy hypothesis in the physical disability field will depend on how much we know about the process of restoring work capacity. It cannot be done from prescriptions based upon a narrow understanding of human productivity.

That challenge persists to this day; many therapists in physical disabilities settings struggle to incorporate occupation-based interventions into their daily work.

Occupational Behavior Model

Mary Reilly is credited as the founder of the **occupational behavior model**. Shannon[21] believed that Reilly's model was the profession's best hope for arresting the process of theoretical derailment. (In occupational therapy, conceptual practice models may also be referred to as *frames of reference*.)

Reilly postulated that humans engaged in occupational role behavior that not only served to organize development at a reductionistic level but also served a broader need for productivity, engagement, and socialization. The express purpose of OT intervention was to allow an individual to learn and practice skills and behaviors that were required of occupational roles, identified as preschooler, student, worker, and retiree. By mobilizing and activating the health aspects of role behavior, people would be able to reengage in occupation following illness, disease, or disability.

As professor of occupational therapy at the University of Southern California, Reilly directed more than 90 graduate student projects. Reilly's students incorporated ideas on motive, competence, and adaptation from noted psychologists.[24,25]

Occupational behavior theory postulates that occupational therapy must meet people's needs through the actualization of competency behaviors. Since humans have inherent drives for causality,[26] intervening at the level of personal volition was a critical aspect of occupational behavior theory. The theory hypothesizes that adaptation occurs at different levels: physical capacity, psychological image, and social worth.[27]

The process by which occupational behavior normally developed involved tasks of role maintenance, role learning, and role relearning.[28] This sequence was supported by a developmental process whereby adult work and recreation patterns were formed in childhood play, arts and crafts, games, and chores. Shannon[29] referred to this as the *play-work process*. Robinson[30] explored this developmental process and suggested that it occurred through a sequential progression of learning about rules, skills, and roles (Figure 3-7).

Florey[31] expanded on these ideas and explained that rules are learned through the acquisition of play behaviors, which were in turn linked to intrinsic motive. Reilly[32] summarized these concepts by explaining that humans engage in play to increase capacities to interact with the environment through exploratory, competency, and achievement behaviors.

Exploratory behaviors involve investigating something previously unknown and are often seen through playful interactions. Competency behaviors involve mastery of a specific task or skill through practice. Achievement behaviors involve the accomplishment of a defined goal that is occupationally relevant for role behavior. Exploratory, competency, and achievement behaviors are considered important for normal development and were hypothesized for use as a powerful tool for rehabilitation (Figure 3-8).

Developmental Process of Occupational Behavior

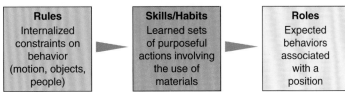

Rules	**Skills/Habits**	**Roles**
Internalized constraints on behavior (motion, objects, people)	Learned sets of purposeful actions involving the use of materials	Expected behaviors associated with a position

Figure 3-7   Occupational behavior is developed through a play-work process rooted in developmental experiences of acquiring skills and habits that translate into learning about rules and role expectations.

Occupational Behavior

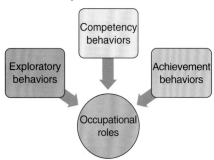

Figure 3-8   Humans interact with the environment and fulfill occupational roles through exploratory, competency, and achievement behaviors.

Model of Human Occupation

Figure 3-9   Gary Kielhofner (Courtesy of the Archive of the American Occupational Therapy Association, Inc.)

Gary Kielhofner (1949-2010; Figure 3-9) was one of Mary Reilly's students. His initial work with occupational behavior theory involved investigating the concept of temporal adaptation and time use.[33] He then began exploring ideas about models related to a general systems theory framework,[34] which informed his thinking about reorganizing occupational behavior constructs into a workable practice model. Many of the concepts worked on by other Reilly students were incorporated into this new model. Kielhofner's **model of human occupation**[35] focuses broadly on volition, habituation, and performance components that support a process of occupational engagement and adaptation. This model will be explored in greater detail in Chapter 4.

Summary

- Habit training is a therapeutic method developed by Eleanor Clarke Slagle and Adolf Meyer aimed at achieving a healthy balance of work, play, rest, and sleep. The patient's daily activities were closely planned, scheduled, and supervised until he or she could assume and maintain those habits on their own.

- Reductionism is a philosophic approach in which complex ideas are understood by breaking them down into smaller parts.

- Science-based methods of practice that focus primarily on correcting physical or mental impairments/disabilities were reductionistic methods based on a medical model.

- Aligning with physician patrons in the early- and mid-20th century provided credibility and security for occupational therapists.

- Early medical leaders of the occupational therapy profession included Adolf Meyer, C. Floyd Haviland, and Joseph Doane.

- Occupational therapists who developed and promoted reductionistic models of practice included Berta Bobath, Margaret Rood, Signe Brunnstrom, A. Jean Ayres, Fern Cramer-Azima, Gail Fidler, and Anne Cronin Mosey.

- A paradigm crisis occurred in the 1970s when many occupational therapists came to believe that the medical model of practice was taking the profession too far away from its original focus on occupation.

- Mary Reilly believed that occupational therapy required a third paradigm, in which the profession reidentified itself as primarily concerned with human occupation. Reilly's occupational behavior model held that humans fulfill their occupational roles by interacting with the environment through exploratory, competency, and achievement behaviors.

- Gary Kielhofner's model of human occupation built on Reilly's occupational behavior premise and focused on volition, habituation, and performance components that support a process of occupational engagement and adaptation.

Reflect and Apply

Individual activity: Think about and record your answers to the following questions

1. How did gender norms in the 20th century impact the developing occupational therapy profession?
2. Why do many modern-day practitioners continue to focus on reductionistic practice models?
3. Occupational therapists frequently use Interest Checklists as an assessment to understand activities or tasks that are important to their patients. What methods might you need to use in different practice settings to learn this information about your patients?

Small group discussion

1. Discuss the pros and cons of reductionistic practice models that were developed by occupational therapy leaders in the 20th century.
2. New billing codes for occupational therapy require the inclusion of an occupational profile as part of an initial assessment. Considering the principles of occupational behavior, what questions would be important to include in any occupational profile? Pair off and practice interviewing techniques to elicit this information.
3. Break into small groups and discuss the concepts of paradigm crisis and paradigm resolution. How do these concepts relate to what have you observed in your initial exposure to occupational therapy practice? Are therapists using occupation as an intervention strategy as well as an outcome objective in the settings you observed? Why or why not?

Review Questions

1. Occupational therapy's first major crisis was the result of pressure to be more

    a. visible.
    b. cost-effective.
    c. scientific.
    d. like physical therapy.

2. In the mechanistic paradigm based on the medical model, occupational therapists

    a. appreciated the importance of occupation in human life.
    b. used occupation as a restorative force.
    c. were primarily concerned with the client factors needed to perform a task.
    d. viewed people in terms of their motivation and desire to participate in meaningful activities.

3. When a profession changes its focus to a new set of values and beliefs, this process is known as a(n)

    a. paradigm shift.
    b. scientific investigation.
    c. example of reductionism.
    d. developmental model.

4. A period of "normal science" in a discipline is marked by

    a. paradigm shifts.
    b. interdisciplinary collaboration.
    c. isolationism.
    d. hypothesis testing.

5. Reductionism is best defined as

    a. eliminating smaller concepts to understand general ideas.
    b. normal science.
    c. breaking complex ideas into smaller concepts.
    d. simplifying a complex hierarchy.

6. Which of the following was an important and beneficial impact of reductionistic practice models in occupational therapy?

    a. Persistent alignment with original core values of OT
    b. Acceptance of OT by medical professionals
    c. Reduced confusion about the OT scope of practice
    d. Expansion of service delivery into nonmedical contexts

7. Which of the following was a negative impact of reductionistic practice models in occupational therapy?

   a. Proliferation of occupational therapy service in institutions
   b. Lack of legitimacy and alignment with medical practice
   c. Unscientific approaches were regarded as "quackery"
   d. Devaluing of principles associated with the Arts and Crafts Movement

8. Which theory states that rules, skills, and roles are learned through a developmental play-work process?

   a. Occupational behavior (Reilly)
   b. Cognitive (Piaget)
   c. Surplus energy (Schiller-Spencer)
   d. Psychodynamic (Roe)

9. The central premise of the occupational behavior model is that

   a. occupational therapy's major task is to prevent and reduce illness.
   b. the occupational therapy profession needs to narrow its sphere for client engagement.
   c. man is malleable and, thus, adaptable to occupational therapy intervention.
   d. man through the use of his hands as they are engaged by his mind and will, can influence the state of his own health.

10. Which of the following best defines occupational behavior?

    a. Includes activities that occupy a person's time, involve achievement, and address the economic realities of life
    b. Addresses the employability of the client
    c. Refers to the specific tasks one must accomplish to achieve full recognition as an adult worker
    d. Refers to the developmental continuum inherent in childhood play

11. In the current paradigm, occupational therapy practitioners believe that

    a. a person's quality of life is based on biologic well-being.
    b. being meaningfully occupied is fundamental to well-being.
    c. disease eradication is of major concern to the occupational therapy profession.
    d. one of the profession's mandates is to solve problems that threaten survival.

12. Reilly explicitly stated that it was important for occupational therapists to focus on which of the following?

    a. Exploration, competency, and achievement behaviors
    b. Psychosexual and familial role behaviors
    c. Spiritual and creatively expressive behaviors
    d. Competitive, ambitious, and goal-oriented work behaviors

References

1. Reilly M. Occupational therapy can be one of the great ideas of 20th century medicine. *Am J Occup Ther*. 1962;16:2-9.
2. Meyer A. The philosophy of occupational therapy. *Arch Occup Ther*. 1922;1:1-10.
3. Peloquin SM. Occupational therapy service: individual and collective understandings of the founders, Part 2. *Am J Occup Ther*. 1991;45:733-744.
4. Kielhofner G. *Conceptual Foundations of Occupational Therapy Practice*. Philadelphia, PA: FA Davis Publisher; 2009.
5. Andersen LT, Reed KL. *The History of Occupational Therapy: The First Century*. Thorofare, NJ: Slack Inc; 2017.
6. Colman W. Structuring education: development of the first educational standards in occupational therapy, 1917-1930. *Am J Occup Ther*. 1992;46(7):653-660.
7. Doane JC. Methods of acquainting the medical profession with the value of occupational therapy. *Occup Ther Rehab*. 1931;10:13-23.
8. Doane JC. Presidential address. (Given at the 15th Annual meeting of AOTA in Toronto, Canada). *Occup Ther Rehab*. 1931;10:363-368.
9. Peters CO. Powerful occupational therapists: a community of professionals, 1950-1980. *Occup Ther Mental Health*. 2011;27(3-4):199-410. doi:10.1080/0164212X.2011.597328.
10. Bobath B. The importance of the reduction of muscle tone and the control of mass reflex action in the treatment of spasticity. *Occup Ther Rehab*. 1948;27(5):371-383.
11. Rood M. Neurophysiological mechanisms utilized in the treatment of neuromuscular dysfunction. *Am J Occup Ther*. 1956;10:220-225.
12. Twitchell TE. The restoration of motor function following hemiplegia in man. *Brain*. 1951;74:443-480.
13. Brunnstrom S. *Movement Therapy in Hemiplegia*. New York, NY: Harper and Row Publishing Co; 1970.
14. Ayres AJ. *Sensory Integration and Learning Disorders*. Los Angeles, CA: Western Psychological Services; 1972.
15. Fiorentino M. *Reflex Testing Methods for Evaluating CNS Development*. Springfield, IL: Charles C. Thomas Publisher; 1963.
16. Moore JC. Behavior, bias, and the limbic system. *Am J Occup Ther*. 1976;30(1):11-19.
17. Azima H, Azima F. Outline of a dynamic theory of occupational therapy. *Am J Occup Ther*. 1959;13:1-7.
18. Azima FJC. The Azima battery: an overview. In: Hemphill BJ, ed. *The Evaluative Process in Psychiatric Occupational Therapy*. Thorofare, NJ: Slack Inc; 1982.
19. Fidler GS, Fidler JW. *Introduction to Psychiatric Occupational Therapy*. New York, NY: Macmillan Publishing Co; 1958.
20. Fidler G, Fidler J. *Occupational Therapy: A Communicative Process in Psychiatry*. New York, NY: Macmillan Publishing Co; 1963.
21. Shannon P. The derailment of occupational therapy. *Am J Occup Ther*. 1977;31(4):229-234.
22. Kuhn TS. *The Structure of Scientific Revolutions*. Chicago, IL: University of Chicago Press; 1962.
23. Hammell KW. Resisting theoretical imperialism in the disciplines of occupational science and occupational therapy. *Br J Occup Ther*. 2011;74(1):27-33.
24. Smith MB. Competence and adaptation. *Am J Occup Ther*. 1974;28:11-15.
25. White RW. The urge towards competence. *Am J Occup Ther*. 1971;25:271-274.
26. Burke JP. A clinical perspective on motivation: pawn versus origin. *Am J Occup Ther*. 1977;31:254-258.
27. Heard C. Occupational role acquisition: a perspective on the chronically disabled. *Am J Occup Ther*. 1977;31:243-247.
28. Matsutsuyu J. Occupational behavior: a perspective on work and play. *Am J Occup Ther*. 1971;25:291-294.

29. Shannon P. The work-play model: a basis for occupational therapy programming in psychiatry. *Am J Occup Ther*. 1970;24:215-218.
30. Robinson A. Play: the arena for acquisition of rules for competent behavior. *Am J Occup Ther*. 1977;31:248-253.
31. Florey L. An approach to play and play development. *Am J Occup Ther*. 1971;26:275-280.
32. Reilly M. *Play as Exploratory Learning*. Beverly Hills, CA: Sage Publications; 1974.
33. Kielhofner G. Temporal adaptation: a conceptual framework for occupational therapy. *Am J Occup Ther*. 1977;31:235-242.
34. Kielhofner G. General systems theory: implications for theory and action in occupational therapy. *Am J Occup Ther*. 1978;32:637-645.
35. Kielhofner G, Burke JP. A model of human occupation, part 1. Conceptual framework and content. *Am J Occup Ther*. 1980;34:572-581.
36. West WL. Ten milestone issues in AOTA history. *Am J Occup Ther*. 1992;46:1066-1074.

two

Theory-Driven Approaches to Practice

4 Modern Occupation-Based Approaches

Occupation is the purposeful use of time by humans to fulfill their own internal urges toward exploring and mastering their environment that at the same time fulfills the requirements of the social group to which they belong and personal needs for self-maintenance.

—Gary Kielhofner[1]

Chapter Outline

Learning Objectives

1. Explain what is meant by the term *occupation-based model*.
2. Identify modern occupation-based approaches.
3. State the key principles of person–environment–occupation models.
4. State the key principles of the ecology of the human performance model.
5. State the key principles of the occupational adaptation model.

6. Determine the prevalence of occupation-based models in clinical practice.
7. Explain why a practice framework was developed by the American Occupational Therapy Association.

Key Terms

ecology of human performance model
habituation
occupational adaptation
occupational adaptation model
occupational performance
performance capacity
person–environment–occupation models
volition

Overview

Research indicates that the model of human occupation (MOHO), descended from the ideas of Mary Reilly and her graduate students, is the most broadly used occupation-based practice model. Other occupation-based models are used by smaller numbers of clinicians. This "occupation-based" concept has been widely accepted within the occupational therapy community. During the 20th century, academic theoreticians developed a new lexicon based on a renewed interest in occupational concepts, and clinicians understood that occupation-based models differed from reductionistic models of practice.

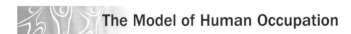

The Model of Human Occupation

Dr Gary Kielhofner is the primary author of MOHO, although many others contributed to his work over time. Reed[2] identifies MOHO as a "third generation model in occupational therapy." As we saw in Chapter 3, the original philosophies of Adolph Meyer and Eleanor Clark Slagle provided the foundation for Reilly's occupational behavior model,[3] which in turn was foundational for MOHO.

MOHO is unique to occupational therapy but incorporates ideas from other disciplines. The purpose of this model is to provide a framework for clinicians to understand how patients choose occupations, develop habits and routines, and ultimately perform within a larger environment[4] (see Table 4-1). These processes develop and occur through the interaction of several important factors. MOHO describes three human subsystems (volitional, habituation, and performance capacity) and their relationships to occupation and the environment (Figure 4-1). Each of these subsystems contributes different but complementary aspects to the occupational behavior of every individual.

Table 4-1
Model of Human Occupation (MOHO)

THEORY AND KEY READINGS	DEFINING FUNCTION	DEFINING DYSFUNCTION	ASSESSMENT	INTERVENTION
Influenced by the original occupational behavior work at the University of Southern California and Gary Kielhofner's master's thesis, which was refined by Burke and Igi.[1,18-20]	Healthy and competent performance in occupations of self-care, work, and play that contributes to balance and role fulfillment.	The inability to perform occupations or an interruption in role performance leading to decreased quality of life.	Assessment data are used to frame the patient's challenge and to guide clinical reasoning and goal setting. Tools include: • MOHOST—assesses capacity for occupational functioning • COSA—assesses a child's perception of competence in ADL • Interest Checklist—assesses interests and activity participation over time • AMPS—assesses motor and process skills related to functional performance in specific tasks • Role Checklist—assesses adult role behavior	• Intended to promote self-organization through participation in occupation. • Considers the impact of the environment on all aspects of human functioning. • Directed at identified problems in volition, habituation, and performance systems based on assessment results. • Intervention outcomes are expected to primarily impact occupational identity and occupational role performance.

Abbreviations: ADL, activities of daily living; AMPS, assessment of motor and process skills; COSA, Children's Occupational Self-Assessment; MOHOST, MOHO Screening Tool.

Volitional System

Volition is the power to make a choice or decision. The volitional system is the motivation for human action. An individual's personality and experiences influence whether his or her actions are more intrinsically or extrinsically directed. For example, a young child with cerebral palsy may come to rely on caregivers to provide assistance to move and play with toys. This may reinforce elements of an external locus of control for the child. However, a person's values and interests also influence their motive to act. In this example, the child's parents may notice that including an older sibling in play activities is reinforcing and motivating to the child, encouraging a desire to move more independently. This may reinforce elements of an internal locus of control for the child. The combination of these factors must be carefully considered by the occupational therapist in regard to their impact on an individual's

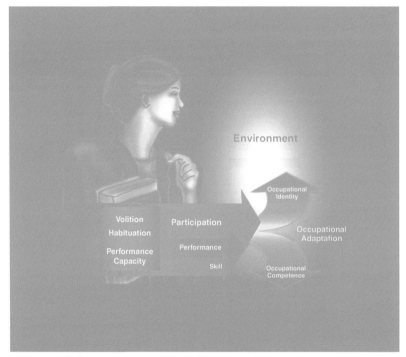

Figure 4-1   Key concepts of the model of human occupation. (Reprinted with permission from Kielhofner G. *Model of Human Occupation: Theory and Application*. 4th ed. Baltimore, MD: Lippincott Williams & Wilkins; 2007.)

functioning. Therapists consider a person's existing volitional system and also evaluate how to help him or her activate a desire for occupational participation. Successful therapists are highly skilled in understanding the dynamics of their patient's volitional systems.

Habituation System

Habituation is the process of becoming used to something or of establishing routines. The habituation system is an organizing system for human activity. Habits are routine and automatic actions that make up important and meaningful components of our daily lives. Habits are further expressed through role behavior, which serves as a construct of our inner identity and also as a structure for our interaction with others. For example, a young father previously enjoyed running as a leisure activity but now finds that the demands of parenting often interfere with his daily running habit. Running and other fitness activities were such an important element of his identity that he could not just end his participation once his child was born. When his daughter became old enough to ride in a jogging stroller, he was able to include her in his running routine. Successful therapists understand the importance of the habituation system. When life changes occur, clinicians can often help people develop new routines that will support both occupational role and identity.

Performance Capacity

Performance capacity refers to the physical and mental processes and abilities that underlie the performance of an activity. For example, grandmother diagnosed with congestive heart failure has physical limitations in strength and endurance that impact her ability to provide after-school care for her grandchildren. She also experiences anxiety because of her fragile health status and how her condition limits her ability to be an effective caregiver. This woman's problems with physical endurance and anxiety are important to understand in the context of her illness and also in the context of her sense of personal competency and ability to engage in valued occupations. MOHO helps to move a clinician's thinking beyond a reductionistic perspective that focuses only on symptoms and toward a more expansive understanding of how these problems influence human occupation.

Environment

MOHO defines the environment as specific physical, social, cultural, economic, and political features of the particular contexts within which we live.[4] Each element of a person's environment provides opportunities, resources, demands, and constraints. How we feel or notice these and how (or whether) they influence our occupational behavior depends on each person's volition, habituation, and performance capacity (see Figure 4-1). For example, the degree of independence that might be required of a person to complete self-care routines is strongly influenced by environmental factors. A teenager is expected to be able to independently change into a swimsuit for physical education class, but that same skill would not be expected of an adult in a skilled nursing facility without swimming activities or aquatic therapy. Also note that preferred leisure activities and patterns may vary depending on the cultural values of specific ethnic groups. The influence of environmental factors on human occupation is pervasive and important for therapists to consider when planning interventions.

CASE 4-1   *James (Part 1)*

James is a 38-year-old man. At age 10, he sustained a closed head injury when kicked by a horse. When asked about the incident, all he remembers is playing on his uncle's farm and climbing a fence to get a better look at the horses. He has no memory of his injury. Throughout his teen years, he received rehabilitation services.

James recounts growing up in a small town and enjoying his summer job as an activities assistant, helping residents in a nursing facility. When he was 22, he moved to a large city, where he currently resides. He began experiencing mental health problems after the move, when he was in a stressful job. He experienced delusional thoughts and was in and out of the hospital several times.

At the present time, he can negotiate daily activities but has a mild right hemiparesis and perseveration and has problems with speech articulation and short-term memory. He lives an isolated life in a supervised group home with three other men. His family lives far away. Faced with large expanses of time, he often retreats to his bed or obsessively writes to organize his thoughts and ward off feelings of emptiness and loneliness. James fiercely values being independent.

In the past, James participated in supervised work programs. A recent vocational rehabilitation assessment suggested that he was ready to work in a transitional setting. Anxious to work to feel useful and earn enough money to move to his own apartment, he agreed with his vocational counselor's plans for him to work at a new cooperative business. James worked as part of a furniture production line with 30 other people who have persistent mental illness. After 6 months, he was referred to an occupational therapist for assessment and consultation, because he was not satisfied with working at the cooperative, and staff reported that he was not fitting in.

Using the theoretical foundations, concepts, and assumptions inherent in MOHO:

1. Describe the nature of the patient–therapist relationship between James and this occupational therapist.
2. List the questions the occupational therapist would ask as part of assessing James's assets and liabilities, skills, and the influences of the environment on his occupational behavior.
3. Describe intervention strategies that the occupational therapist might use to minimize James's problems and achieve his occupational goals.
4. Describe the expected outcome of the occupational therapy intervention process.

Person–Environment–Occupation Models

Several models share common elements that focus on the transactional relationship between the person, the environment, and the occupations being performed. All the **person–environment–occupation (PEO) models** define the person as a sum of mind, body, and spiritual components. The environment is defined as in MOHO. All PEO models maintain that people have variable values, interests, skills, and experiences that influence occupational performance (see Table 4-2). **Occupational performance** is defined as the ability to complete a task that is related to self-care, productivity, or leisure participation. The terms *activities*, *tasks*, and *occupations* are used to describe actions performed by humans; full consensus on these terms has not been achieved.[5]

The PEO models share common assumptions:

- A top-down approach to clinical problem solving is recommended.
- People are unique and should be treated as autonomous agents.
- People engage in a variety of tasks (occupations).
- Environments are complex and should be considered in broad terms.

Table 4-2
Person–Environment–Occupation (PEO) Models

THEORY AND KEY READINGS	DEFINING FUNCTION	DEFINING DYSFUNCTION	ASSESSMENT	INTERVENTION
PEO models share common elements that were identified in basic ecologic theories, including a systems-focus on the interaction of personal, environmental, and other factors in human performance.[6-8]	At the most basic level, defined as a *goodness of fit* between person, environmental, and occupational factors.	Dysfunction occurs when personal capacities (intrinsic) or environmental barriers (extrinsic) limit performance in occupations and engagement.	Framed in terms of what is most important to the person, as determined through various tools: • COPM for adults • CAPE/PAC • Additional personal-level and task/occupation assessments can be included, as well as environmental observations.	• Occupation can be used as a medium for improving personal (intrinsic) factors that impede occupational performance. • Modifications to the environment can be made to enable occupational performance and engagement.

Abbreviations: CAPE/PAC, Children's Assessment of Participation and Enjoyment and the Preferred Activities of Children; COPM, Canadian Occupational Performance Measure.

- People impact and are impacted by their environment.
- The transaction between the elements of person, occupation, and environment dictate competence in occupational performance.

A top-down approach to clinical problem solving means that the occupational therapist starts the assessment process by identifying what occupations the person needs or wants to perform. Functionally, PEO approaches have sometimes been difficult to implement in clinical settings that are focused primarily on medical, educational, or developmental outcomes.

PEO models focus on patient autonomy, the value of inclusion, and the confluence of factors that impact occupational performance. All people are considered unique occupational beings interacting within complex environments that can sometimes hinder and sometimes promote performance.

The basic PEO model described by Law et al[6] includes these common elements. Similarly, constructed models include the person–environment–occupation–performance model (PEOP)[7] that continues to be developed and periodically updated (Figure 4-2).

Both PEO and PEOP state that behavior cannot be separated from contextual influences and that people express occupational performance developmentally across time. The notion of *fit* between elements is important in understanding a person's performance. A widely cited PEO model[8] is illustrated in Figure 4-3. This model is now commonly referred to as the Canadian model of occupational performance and engagement (CMOP-E).

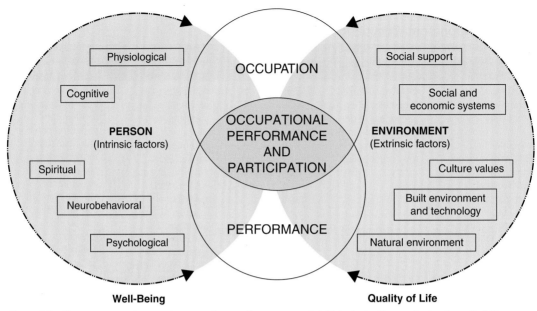

Figure 4-2   The person–environment–occupation–performance model. (Adapted with permission from Christiansen C, Baum C, Bass-Haugen J, eds. *Occupational Therapy: Performance, Participation, and Well-Being*. 3rd ed. Thorofare, NJ: Slack Inc; 2005.)

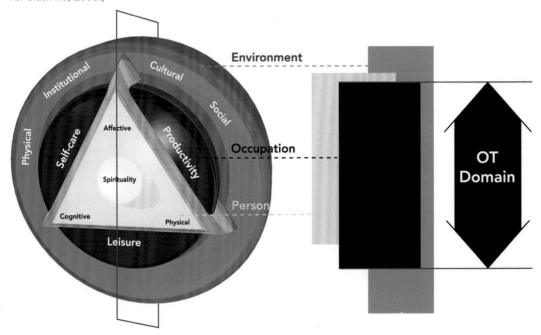

Figure 4-3   The Canadian model of occupational performance and engagement. OT, occupational therapy. (Reprinted with permission from Potalko HJ, Townsend EA, Craik J. Canadian model of occupational performance and engagement (CMOP-E). In: Townsend EA, Polatajko HJ, eds. *Enabling Occupation II: Advancing an Occupational Therapy Vision of Health, Well-being, & Justin through Occupation*. Ottawa, ON: CAOT Publications ACE; 2007.)

The initial expressions of PEO models focused on the transactional relationships between personal, environmental, and occupational elements. Later iterations (PEOP and CMOP-E) included a stronger focus on participation in meaningful occupations, engagement with others and society, and spirituality.

CASE 4-1   *James (Part 2)*

Using the theoretical foundations, concepts, and assumptions inherent in PEO models:

1. Describe the nature of the patient/therapist relationship between James and this occupational therapist.
2. List some questions the occupational therapist could ask to identify James's concerns. Describe what data the occupational therapist would gather regarding personal and environmental factors.
3. Describe the intervention strategies that the occupational therapist might use to improve the fit between James's ability and his preferred occupations, given his current context.
4. Describe the expected outcome of the occupational therapy intervention process.

Ecology of Human Performance Model

The **ecology of human performance (EHP) model** (Figure 4-4) was designed with the purpose of accounting for the influence of the environment on human performance. Based on the assumption that "occupational therapy is most effective when it is imbedded in real life,"[9] temporal and environmental contextual factors are identified that allow practitioners to interpret behavior and choose appropriate and meaningful therapeutic interventions (see Table 4-3). This approach raises important questions about the subjective nature of contextual relevance and concerns about the validity of standardized assessment tools that provide information without context.

Occupations, by their very nature, are interpreted in light of contextual meaning. Without this saturation of meaning, occupations are reduced to simple, robotic tasks. While on an extended work experience as a visiting scholar in another country, Hasselkus[10] describes her experiences of feeling stripped of her occupations while immersed in an unfamiliar culture with unfamiliar routines. Deprived of her familiar context, she began to question her own identity. She states that her ability to participate in even simple but familiar routines provided a grounding foundation for her other experiences. She held that occupational therapy could be a powerful and normalizing force by helping to reestablish habits and routines after a significant disruption in a person's life.

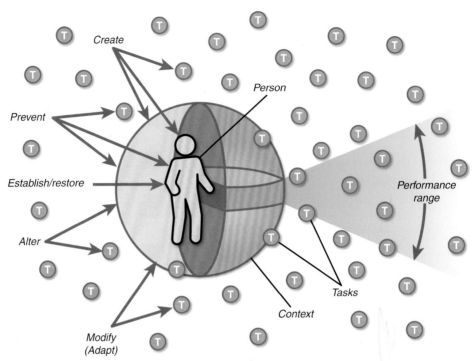

Figure 4-4   The ecology of human performance model. T, tasks. (Reprinted with permission from Dunn W, McClain LH, Brown C, Youngstrom MJ. The ecology of human performance. In: Crepeau EB, Cohn ES, Schell BAB, eds. *Willard & Spackman's Occupational Therapy*. 10th ed. Philadelphia, PA: Lippincott Williams & Wilkins; 2003: 223-226.)

The EHP model emphasizes the importance of considering contextual factors in intervention. It also delineates specific approaches that occupational therapists might take. This model holds that occupational therapists engage in different levels of intervention planning focused on an understanding of the person's engagement of tasks within different contexts.

Consider a person with a recent hip replacement. The first intervention option is to establish or restore contextually relevant skills and abilities. For example, an occupational therapist might help this patient learn lower-extremity dressing skills following the surgery.

The second option is to alter the performance context. In this example, a home health aide could come to the person's home after discharge to provide assistance with completing cooking and self-care tasks.

A third option is to adapt contextual features to support performance. For example, temporary changes to the home could be made, such as using a tub transfer bench to get in and out of the shower.

A fourth option is to prevent negative outcomes. Since the patient may have increased risk of falls, the occupational therapist might suggest removing throw rugs or increasing illumination.

A fifth option is to create more adaptable performance in context. For example, the occupational therapist might encourage normal role participation by finding ways for the person to still attend church and participate in other meaningful social activities.

Table 4-3
Ecology of Human Performance (EHP) Model

THEORY AND KEY READINGS	DEFINING FUNCTION	DEFINING DYSFUNCTION	ASSESSMENT	INTERVENTION
The EHP model was developed by Winnie Dunn and occupational therapy faculty at the University of Kansas Medical Center.[9]	When the environment or context matches a person's abilities so that they can engage in tasks.	An unbalanced relationship between the person, the task, and the environment that impairs performance.	• No specific evaluations are required. • Therapists are encouraged to assess with skilled observations of occupational performance in relevant environments.	Therapists should choose from the following strategies to promote occupational performance: • Establish/restore (remediate person's skills/abilities). • Alter the actual context in which person performs. • Adapt contextual features and/or task demands to support performance in context. • Prevent the occurrence or evolution of maladaptive performance. • Create circumstances that promote more adaptable or complex performance in context.

CASE 4-1   *James (Part 3)*

Using the theoretical foundations, concepts, and assumptions inherent in the EHP model:

1. Describe the nature of the patient–therapist relationship between James and this occupational therapist.
2. List the questions the occupational therapist would ask to identify and incorporate James's life context.
3. Describe the intervention strategies that the occupational therapist might use to:
   a. Establish/restore James's skills/abilities
   b. Alter the actual context in which he performs
   c. Adapt contextual features and/or task demands to support his performance in the context of that performance

     d. Prevent the occurrence or evolution of maladaptive performance in James's life

     e. Create circumstances that promote adaptable or complex performance in his context.

  4. Describe the expected outcome of the occupational therapy intervention process.

Occupational Adaptation Model

The **occupational adaptation (OA) model** (Figure 4-5) is an occupation-based model that was designed to describe both the state and the process of OA (see Table 4-4). **Occupational adaptation** is a normal process that "exists in humans to allow us to respond masterfully and adaptively to the various occupational challenges that we encounter over a lifetime."[11] OA is seen as a normal process that occurs in people of all ages; however, it is sometimes at risk during periods of transition or stress.

    Many aspects of this model are similar to other occupation-based models except that the focus is on the process of adaptation itself. The model states that people are occupational

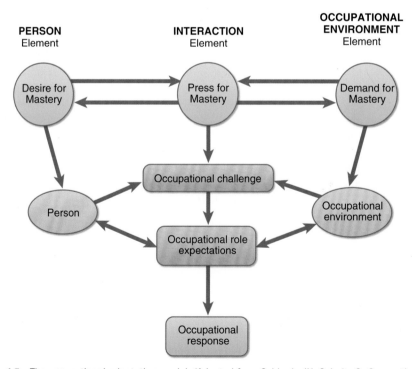

Figure 4-5   The occupational adaptation model. (Adapted from Schkade JK, Schultz S. Occupational adaptation: Toward a holistic approach to contemporary practice, Part 1. *Am J Occup Ther.* 1992;46:829-837.)

Table 4-4
Occupational Adaptation (OA) Model

THEORY AND KEY READINGS	DEFINING FUNCTION	DEFINING DYSFUNCTION	ASSESSMENT	INTERVENTION
The concept of OA was selected by Texas Woman's University as a focus for research and to guide intervention.[11,21,22]	A person's ability to make adaptive changes so that they can function in a way that is efficient, effective, and satisfying to self and others.	When there are environmental demands that cannot be met and that cause subsequent occupational challenges.	• No specific evaluations are required • Therapists are encouraged to determine roles and environments that are relevant, the environmental demands and the individual's abilities to meet those demands, and to assess for the relative degree of mastery in these contexts.	• Improve patient ability to adapt by improving occupational readiness. • Improve ability to engage in meaningful occupational activities. • The role of the therapist is to pose questions and make observations that will help the individual develop his/her own adaptive responses.

beings with a desire to master the environment and that the environment demands mastery from the person. This transactional relationship between the person and the environment is called the press for mastery, and normative developmental experiences are used to navigate this transaction. Performance problems occur when a person's abilities or resources cannot meet environmental demand. Using this model, the therapist's goal is to facilitate adaptive responses from the individual so that their performance is effective, efficient, and satisfying.

Three primary barriers have been identified that limit the application of this model in a clinical context: a lack of clarity related to the concept of OA, few outcome studies that measure OA, and a lack of specific assessment tools for this model.[12] Despite these limitations, OA constructs are useful as an occupation-based model and will benefit from continued development and refinement.

CASE 4-1   *James (Part 4)*

Using the theoretical foundations, concepts, and assumptions inherent in the OA model:

1. Describe the nature of the patient–therapist relationship between James and this occupational therapist.
2. List the questions the occupational therapist would ask to identify the sources of James's dysfunction, and describe what data the occupational therapist would

gather regarding James's occupational environments, role expectations, and the effect of the presenting problem on James's systems.
3. Describe the intervention strategies that the occupational therapist might use to maximize James's internal adaptation processes and the use of meaningful occupations.
4. Describe the expected outcome of the occupational therapy intervention process.

Comparison and Prevalence of Occupation-Based Models

As we have seen, each occupation-based approach focuses on slightly different elements of an individual's situation, environment, abilities, and disability (if present). Some differences are only a matter of how the presenting problem is framed, although that in itself can influence the direction that intervention might take.

There is a significant overlap among all of these approaches, and the nuances are sometimes difficult to discern without reading the source material closely to understand differences in definitions of terms. Any of these approaches can be useful for the occupational therapist to focus thinking on the broad nature of occupation, even when it is necessary to introduce reductionistic models that address components related to physical, cognitive, or psychosocial functioning. Table 4-5 provides a comparison of occupation-based models.

Prevalence in Practice

Occupational therapy researchers have studied the occupation-based models to determine their validity, relevance, and clinical prevalence. Lee[13] identified 503 published works related to occupation-based models, with 86% of publications relating to MOHO, 6% relating to OA, 5% relating to PEO models, and 3% relating to EHP. She found that MOHO was clearly subjected to the most testing and had the largest research base. Although MOHO was established earlier than the other models, it remains a trending interest of current researchers.

Bent et al[14] reported that in a survey of entry-level practitioners, MOHO was the most commonly reported occupation-based model being used, although the reported use of that model was low. In a survey completed by Lee et al,[15] 81% of practitioners reported using MOHO at least some of the time. The two populations of therapists that were surveyed differed in regard to several important factors (including years of experience and patient population served), and this may have contributed to the different findings.

The absence of any universally accepted occupation-based model contributed to efforts on the part of professional occupational therapy associations to develop their

Table 4-5
Comparison of Occupation-Based Models

MODEL	PATIENT–THERAPIST RELATIONSHIP	ASSESSMENT	INTERVENTION	OUTCOME(S)
MOHO	Interactive Emphasizes the person's individuality The individual participates in identifying problems and setting goals.	Variety of assessment tools are used to evaluate the individual's assets, liabilities, performance, and influence of environment on occupational behavior.	Enable the individual to find a meaningful role in the work setting that he/she can perform well. Use occupations that have meaning to the person to improve his/her skills. Reorganize the work environment to facilitate his skill development	Enable the individual to develop, adapt, and make life transitions. Improved skills and development of new roles and habits
PEO models	Interactive Therapist as an active agent in the person's environment	Identify important occupations. Assess intrinsic and extrinsic factors that impact performance and engagement.	Use occupation as a means to achieve occupational balance between PEOP factors.	Improved fit between personal, environmental, and occupational factors for engagement and quality of life
OA	Interdependent Therapist as an agent within the person's occupational environment. The individual is an agent of his/her unique personal systems.	Identify sources of dysfunction in OA processes, including personal system and occupational environment. Determine match with role expectations.	Improve OA through therapy using occupational readiness and occupational activity.	Improved self-initiation, generalization, and relative mastery
EHP	Collaborative Involves collaboration among the individual, therapist, and staff at work setting.	Evaluate the individual's performance of tasks within the context of the work setting. Consider physical, social, cultural, and temporal features of the environment.	Use a variety of interventions to alter the context of the work setting to enable the individual to perform tasks with his/her current skills. Adapt contextual feature or task. Provide remedial skills training to improve quality and quantity of work.	Enable functional performance to emerge as part of the individual's work (with assigned tasks) and in his/her living situation. Improved match between the individual and the work setting.

Abbreviations: EHP, ecology of human performance; MOHO, model of human occupation; OA, occupational adaptation; PEO, person–environment–occupation; PEOP, person–environment–occupation–performance.

own frameworks to explain and guide practice. These associations recognized that clinical practice was still deeply rooted in reductionistic components, and this was partially reinforced by association documents such as the Uniform Terminology system from the American Occupational Therapy Association (AOTA).[16] Additionally, the terms listed in the Uniform Terminology document and subsequently used by clinicians were not always familiar to external audiences.

These factors contributed to interest in adoption of language from the International Classification of Functioning, Disability and Health (ICF) and the creation of the Occupational Therapy Practice Framework,[17] now in its third edition. The ICF is the World Health Organization's framework for measuring health and disability at both the individual and the population levels. The AOTA Framework has been broadly used as an official association document to outline and explain practice issues. The framework outlines a process for occupational therapy, but most theoreticians do not consider it to be a practice model. So, although it encompasses many elements of occupation-based models, it remains a document subject to periodic revision that has not been researched for validity or prevalence.

Summary

- The purpose of MOHO is to provide a framework for clinicians to understand how patients choose occupations, develop habits and routines, and ultimately perform within a larger environment. According to MOHO, three human subsystems—volitional, habituation, and performance capacity—contribute different but complementary aspects to the occupational behavior of every individual.

- PEO models focus on the transactional relationship between the person, the environment, and the occupations being performed.

- The EHP model aims to account for the influence of the environment on human performance. Temporal and environmental contextual factors are identified that allow practitioners to interpret behavior and choose appropriate therapeutic interventions.

- The focus of the OA model is on the process of adaptation itself. This model states that people are occupational beings who have a desire to master the environment and that the environment demands mastery from the person.

- MOHO is the occupation-based model that has been the most researched; the majority of occupational therapy practitioners report using MOHO at least some of the time.

- The absence of any universally accepted occupation-based model contributed to the development of the AOTA *Practice Framework*, which outlines a process for occupational therapy but is not considered a practice model.

Reflect and Apply

Individual and partner activities

1. Based on observations of occupational therapy practice or field experience, what do you perceive as the primary barriers to clinical use of occupation-based models of practice? What are the experiences of your peers? Write a one-page summary explaining the barriers and propose one or two solutions.
2. Compare and contrast the different occupation-based practice models. Work with a partner to create a side-by-side comparison of what an occupational therapy session might look like if you were using one of these models as opposed to another.

Small-group discussion

1. Break into small groups and discuss the use of the term *occupation-based models of practice*. Do you think that this terminology helps or hurts the profession? Should it be used only for internal conversation, or is it something that should be used to describe the profession's orientation to external stakeholders?
2. Interview one or two occupational therapy practitioners and ask them about their familiarity with and use of the *Occupational Therapy Practice Framework*. Participate in a whole-class or small-group discussion to review everyone's findings. List the reasons why practitioners are or are not using this document in practice.

Review Questions

1. What types of models were developed on the basis of a renewed interest in the core philosophy of the occupational therapy profession?

   a. Occupation-based models
   b. Medical-based models
   c. Education-based models
   d. Arts and crafts–based models

2. In MOHO, volition is most associated with which of the following?

   a. Routine actions
   b. Skills
   c. Personal causation
   d. Roles

3. In MOHO, habituation is most associated with which of the following?

   a. Routine actions
   b. Skills
   c. Personal causation
   d. Roles

4. In MOHO, performance is most associated with which of the following?

   a. Routine actions
   b. Skills
   c. Personal causation
   d. Roles

5. Which of the following is *not* a common assumption in PEO models?

   a. Environment is influential.
   b. Patient autonomy is primary.
   c. Person-level factors are important.
   d. Bottom-up approach is mandatory.

6. In the OA model, the transactional relationship between the person and the environment is called

   a. desire for mastery.
   b. demand for mastery.
   c. press for mastery.
   d. opportunity for mastery.

7. According to several research studies, which occupation-based model is most commonly used by occupational therapy clinicians?

   a. PEO model
   b. OA model
   c. MOHO
   d. Occupational therapy practice framework

8. The Occupational Therapy Practice Framework is best described as a(n)

   a. occupation-based practice model.
   b. document used to discuss and explain occupational therapy practice.
   c. philosophy of the occupational therapy profession.
   d. all of the above.

References

1. Kielhofner G. A model of human occupation, part 2: ontogenesis from the perspective of temporal adaptation. *Am J Occup Ther*. 1980;34:657-663.
2. Reed K. *Models of Practice in Occupational Therapy*. Baltimore, MD: Lippincott Williams & Wilkins; 1984.

3. Reilly M. Occupational therapy can be one of the great ideas of 20th century medicine. *Am J Occup Ther*. 1962;16:1-9.

4. Kielhofner G. *A Model of Human Occupation: Theory and Application*. 4th ed. Baltimore, MD: Lippincott Williams & Wilkins; 2008.

5. Baptiste S. The person-environment-occupation model. In: Hinojosa J, Kramer P, Brasic-Royeen C, eds. *Perspective on Human Occupation: Theories Underlying Practice*. 2nd ed. Philadelphia, PA: FA Davis; 2017:144.

6. Law M, Cooper BA, Strong S, Stewart D, Rigby P, Letts L. The person-environment-occupation model: a transactive approach to occupational performance. *Can J Occup Ther*. 1996;63(1):219-233.

7. Christiansen C. Occupational therapy: intervention for life performance. In: Christiansen C, Baum C eds. *Occupational Therapy: Overcoming Human Performance Deficits*. Thorofare, NJ: Slack Inc; 1991.

8. Polatajko HJ, Townsend EA, Craik J. Canadian model of occupational performance and engagement (CMOP-E). In: Townsend EA, Polatajko HJ, eds. *Enabling Occupation II: Advancing an Occupational Therapy Vision of Health, Well-Being, & Justice Through Occupation*. Ottawa, ON: CAOT Publications ACE; 2007:22-36.

9. Dunn W, Brown C, McGuigan A. The ecology of human performance: a framework for considering the effect of context. *Am J Occup Ther*. 1996;48(1994):595-607.

10. Hasselkus B. Habits of the heart. *Am J Occup Ther*. 2000;54(3):247-248. doi:10.5014/ajot.54.3.247.

11. Schkade JK, McClung M. *Occupational Adaptation in Practice: Concepts and Cases*. Thorofare, NJ: Slack Incorporated; 2001:2.

12. Grajo L, Boisselle A, DaLomba E. Occupational adaptation as a construct: a scoping review of literature. *Open J Occup Ther*. 2018;6(1). doi:10.15453/2168-6408.1400.

13. Lee J. Achieving best practice: a review of evidence linked to occupation-focused practice models. *Occup Ther Health Care*. 2010;24(3):206-222. doi:10.3109/07380577.2010.483270.

14. Bent M, Crist P, Florey L, Strickland L. A practice analysis of occupational therapy and impact on certification examination. *OTJR*. 2005;25(3):105-118.

15. Lee S, Taylor R, Kielhofner G, Fisher G. Theory use in practice: a national survey of therapists who use the Model of Human Occupation. *Am J Occup Ther*. 2008;62(1):106-117.

16. American Occupational Therapy Association. Uniform terminology—third edition: application to practice. *Am J Occup Ther*. 1994;48(11):1055-1059. doi:10.5014/ajot.48.11.1055.

17. American Occupational Therapy Association. Occupational therapy practice framework: domain and process (3rd edition). *Am J Occup Ther*. 2014;68(suppl_1):S1-S48. doi:10.5014/ajot.2014.682006.

18. Kielhofner G. A model of human occupation, part 3: benign and vicious cycles. *Am J Occup Ther*. 1980;34:731-737.

19. Kielhofner G, Burke J. A model of human occupation, part 1: conceptual framework and content. *Am J Occup Ther*. 1980;34:572-581.

20. Kielhofner G, Burke J, Igi CH. A model of human occupation, part 4: assessment and intervention. *Am J Occup Ther*. 1980;34:777-788.

21. Schkade JK, Schultz S. Occupational adaptation: toward a holistic approach for contemporary practice, part 1. *Am J Occup Ther*. 1992;46:829-837.

22. Schultz S, Schkade JK. Occupational adaptation: toward a holistic approach for contemporary practice, part 2. *Am J Occup Ther*. 1992;46:917-925.

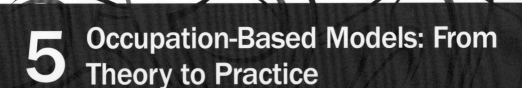

5 Occupation-Based Models: From Theory to Practice

If occupational therapy is to deliver its fullest promise, models of practice in occupational therapy that are exemplary must be identified, applauded, and established as standard bearers for practice everywhere.

—Wendy Wood[1]
American Journal of Occupational Therapy

Chapter Outline

An Eclectic Approach to Practice
Theory As the Basis for Practice
General Systems Theory
   Systems Theory and Occupational Therapy
The NOBA Approach to Practice
Contemporary Clinical Reasoning
Evaluating Approaches and Models of Practice
   Pragmatism

Learning Objectives

1. Describe the value of an eclectic approach to clinical practice and outline the concerns associated with this approach.
2. State the purpose of using theory as the basis for practice.
3. Explain the key principles of general systems theory and how these apply to clinical problem solving.
4. Identify the types of environmental pressures that can influence clinical decision making.

5. Explain how the NOBA approach is used in determining the most appropriate practice model(s) for a specific patient/client.
6. Describe the two major influences on contemporary clinical reasoning.
7. List the steps involved and the questions asked in evaluating possible intervention approaches and models of practice.

Key Terms

biomedical
biosocial
closed system
eclecticism
general systems theory
NOBA method
open system

Overview

This chapter provides a structure for organizing occupational therapy knowledge into a practice model. Many occupational therapists, educators, and students recognize that sometimes there is a philosophical divide between what is espoused as "best practice" and what occurs in the clinical setting. This is not a new problem. Recall Shannon's views on the "derailment" of occupational therapy practice[2] (see Chapter 3) as clinicians focused on reductionistic models of intervention as opposed to occupation-based models that were more expansive and systems based. Although concerns about reductionism were outlined more than 40 years ago, to date, the issue has not been fully resolved.

An Eclectic Approach to Practice

Clinicians report that a lack of unifying theory is a primary barrier to using theory in practice.[3] Ikiugu et al[4] suggested that a solution to the lack of a unifying conceptual foundation is to eclectically combine practice models based on clinical utility.

The term *eclectic* refers to adopting ideas or styles from a broad and diverse range of sources. **Eclecticism** in a therapeutic context is defined as incorporating a variety of therapeutic principles and approaches to create the ideal treatment program for a specific patient. The concept has been explored deeply in the field of psychotherapy, but there is less understanding of how this approach applies in an occupational therapy context.

Although an eclectic approach is often regarded as having value, its use has also been criticized. The eclectic use of conceptual practice models may not be best for facilitating professional coherence and consistency of methodologies. There is potential for incoherence in the articulation of values and approach and for concepts to be misunderstood or misapplied when they are removed from their original context.[5] Additionally, some occupational therapists may claim to use an eclectic approach, when in reality, the term is used when they do not know how to identify the theoretical models being used.[6(p382)]

Ikiugu et al[4] suggested a framework that involves identifying the relevant and complementary models of practice and changing or adapting them when it is clinically appropriate to do so. This method was endorsed by Wong and Fisher,[7] but those authors also suggest that there are limitations when using this approach with occupation-based models because of nuanced technical differences in the way that various theorists have framed their assumptions and concepts. Similarly, Boniface[8(p27)] states that "there would seem to be absolutely nothing wrong with eclecticism as long as the therapist claiming to be eclectic understands the theory behind the different approaches they are dipping into." However, she also warns that eclecticism can appear to be a lack of understanding if the models are not used under an "umbrella" of a broader occupational therapy theory.

Theory As the Basis for Practice

Clinicians sometimes avoid the use of theory to guide decision making and often default to pragmatic demands to guide practice. For example, in hospitals and nursing facilities, therapists use the Functional Independence Measure (FIM) to assess the functional status of patients during the rehabilitation process. Scores are used to evaluate improvement and the ability to be transferred to the next level of care. In educational settings, therapists define improvement in terms of meeting needs within the primary context of educational relevance.

Neither approach lives up to the "magnificent purpose" of Mary Reilly's vision for the profession (Reilly, 1962) or the purpose of the model of human occupation (the most commonly used occupation-based model), which aims to provide the profession with a "universal conceptual foundation to shape its identity and guide its practice."[9] Occupational therapists need to use a coherent and epistemologically sound theory to direct their practice and avoid basing practice decisions on limited contexts.

Convenient solutions found within specific practice settings may serve an immediate, survival-oriented purpose. However, these solutions have the potential to negatively impact our profession's ability to provide care that is valid, research-based, and promoted to the public as a unique service.

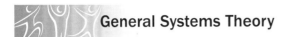

General Systems Theory

General systems theory (GST) originated with biologist Ludwig von Bertalanffy, who first presented the theory in the late 1940s.[10] Its central ideas are that a system is made up of parts that interact to form a coherent whole and that complex systems share organizing principles. In addition to biology, systems theory (also known as systems science) has been applied in the fields of mathematics, psychology, sociology, and business. Kenneth Boulding, an economist and social scientist whose work built on von Bertalanffy's founding principles, also wrote extensively about systems theory.[11]

GST encouraged scientists to turn away from increasingly narrower ranges of focus that limited interdisciplinary communication and collaboration. The basic assumptions of GST are that

- systems are characterized by the dynamic interactions of their components.
- those interactions can be complex and multidirectional.

Although von Bertalanffy and Boulding are not routinely cited in the occupational therapy literature, their contributions to changes in scientific thinking are relevant to occupational therapy's movement away from strictly reductionistic approaches toward a more holistic approach based on individual context and occupation-based models of practice.

Systems Theory and Occupational Therapy

Kielhofner[12] described the principles of GST to the occupational therapy community. He focused particularly on the concept of open systems as an important method for understanding human interactions with the environment. **Open systems** are those that interact with other systems and/or with the outside environment. In contrast, **closed systems** have little or no interaction with other systems or the environment. Humans are considered an open system because of the many levels of interaction within the human body and between individuals and the outside world (Figure 5-1).

Kielhofner was interested in how these interactions relate to occupational role and performance. He expanded on these ideas in introducing his model of human occupation. GST, embedded within this model, provides a framework for inclusive thinking beyond reductionism. Occupational therapists need to focus at multiple levels of systems to understand an individual's occupational functioning.

Without expansive thinking, clinicians may miss important information that is needed to develop the best treatment plan. A nursing home resident is not the sum total of his or her FIM scores. A student is not solely defined by his or her standardized test scores. Systems theory helps us understand that the world is expansive. It encourages us to avoid a tendency to allow limited or survival-oriented thinking to drive our decision making.

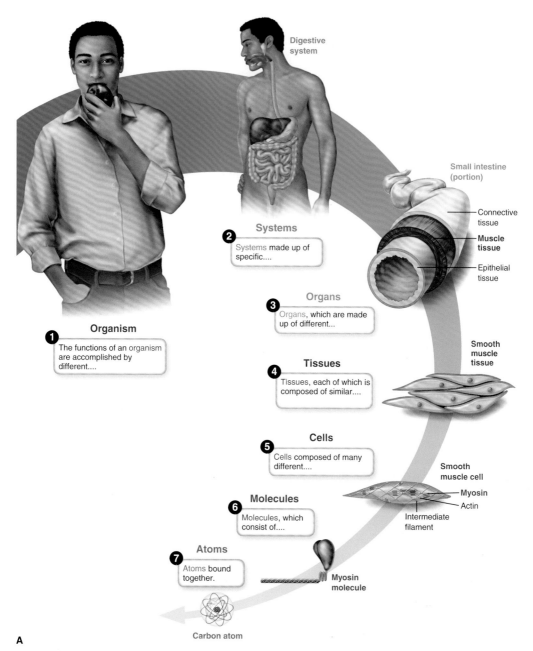

Digestive system

Small intestine (portion)

Connective tissue

Muscle tissue

Epithelial tissue

Systems

2 Systems made up of specific....

Organs

3 Organs, which are made up of different...

Smooth muscle tissue

Organism

1 The functions of an organism are accomplished by different....

Tissues

4 Tissues, each of which is composed of similar....

Cells

5 Cells composed of many different....

Smooth muscle cell

Myosin

Actin

Intermediate filament

Molecules

6 Molecules, which consist of....

Atoms

7 Atoms bound together.

Myosin molecule

Carbon atom

A

Figure 5-1   A, Levels of organization of the human body. B, Levels of systems in human experience based on general systems theory. (A, Reprinted with permission from McConnell TH, Hull KL. *Human Form, Human Function: Essentials of Anatomy & Physiology*. Philadelphia, PA: Lippincott Williams & Wilkins; 2010.)

**General Systems Theory:
Levels of Systems**

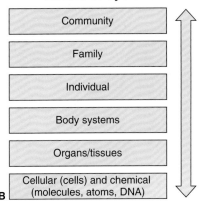

Figure 5-1   *(Continued)*

The NOBA Approach to Practice

The values of occupational therapy's first paradigm in the early 20th century focused on health, skill development, and occupation at a **biosocial** level, involving both biologic and social factors. Several decades later, the values of the second paradigm focused on internal systems, pathology, and symptom reduction at a **biomedical** level. The biomedical approach was primarily focused on addressing physical and mental/emotional impairments and problems. Reilly[13] attempted to resolve these differing orientations in her Occupational Behavior model, outlined in her 1961 Slagle lecture. In this model, she promoted the concept that clinicians should *not only* focus on biomedical or reductionistic science, *but also* remember to attend to biosocial concerns. She referred to this as the **NOBA method** (Figure 5-2). As described in Chapter 3, the

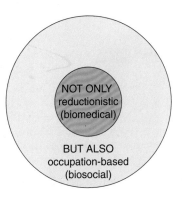

Figure 5-2   Reilly's NOBA method is a holistic approach that requires occupational therapists to *not only* focus on biomedical concerns, *but also* attend to the patient's biosocial needs and concerns.

third paradigm included systems-level thinking, leading to the profession's return to a focus on occupation while incorporating the knowledge associated with treating conditions that impact human performance. This was formalized in Kielhofner's model of human occupation, but the NOBA concept can be just as easily applied with other occupation-based models.

The point of the NOBA method is not where one starts in the process (top down vs bottom up). Instead, this approach emphasizes occupational therapy's unique focus on the range of impact throughout multiple systems. Different clinical situations will dictate different approaches, and occupational therapists should determine which method or methods are best in each situation.[14]

CASE 5-1   *Mary*

An occupational therapist working in an acute care hospital receives a referral for Mary, a 74-year-old woman admitted for pneumonia and exacerbation of chronic obstructive pulmonary disease. Mary has a history of rheumatoid arthritis and type 1 diabetes. The doctor is uncertain if she should be sent home or to a short-term acute rehabilitation facility. During a bedside screen, the therapist notes that Mary becomes short of breath and is unable to safely ambulate 10 feet to the bathroom. She is also unable to participate in her diabetes self-management routines. Upon further assessment, the therapist learns that the patient is recently widowed, lives alone, and has very few social contacts (Figure 5-3).

Analysis

A therapist using a NOBA method will consider all aspects of Mary's condition, from medical concerns to the supports and resources she has access to in the community. The acute care hospital setting may direct the therapist's immediate actions toward biomedical concerns, but the therapist should continually work toward biosocial goals that have meaning and relevance to the patient.

The effective occupational therapist considers all aspects of the patient's situation and problem to understand how to engage the patient in a plan that will lead to greater independence and possible return home. The therapist should have significant concern about how Mary is coping with the recent loss of her husband and about her ability to manage household tasks, given her fragile medical status and lack of social supports. While keeping these concerns in mind, there is a pressing need to determine if Mary can potentially go home. Immediate attention must be paid to bolstering her activity tolerance, strength, and endurance for basic activities of daily living (ADL).

In this situation, the therapist must pay immediate attention to biomedical concerns, while remaining aware and ready to direct attention to more occupation-based concerns once Mary's physical condition stabilizes. The effective occupational therapist is able to formulate a relevant discharge plan that can continue occupational therapy services with a different focus once the treatment setting changes.

1. If the therapist fails to address both biomedical and biosocial issues with this patient, what difficulties might Mary face when she is discharged from the hospital and returns home?
2. Why would an exclusive focus on improving Mary's physical functioning not be the best treatment plan?
3. Why would model of human occupation or another occupation-based model be an excellent choice to guide assessment and intervention planning for this patient?
4. How does the recent loss of Mary's husband affect the approach the therapist might use in this case?

CASE 5-2   *Alyssa*

An occupational therapist working in an outpatient facility receives a referral for Alyssa, a 16-year old with complex regional pain syndrome following an ankle sprain. Alyssa has also been diagnosed with Crohn's disease. During the initial evaluation, the therapist learns that the patient has been using crutches and wearing a controlled ankle motion walking boot for 2 months. Her foot is mildly swollen and her skin is mottled; she complains of 8/10 pain and will not even let her mother touch her foot. The occupational therapist also learns that Alyssa is no longer participating in gymnastics or dance and has missed 50% of school this year because of chronic stomach pain (Figure 5-4).

Analysis

In this situation, the therapist has significant concerns about Alyssa's pain, noting that the ankle condition has persisted for 2 months and the stomach pain is chronic. Since this patient is so hyperresponsive to pain, the therapist decides that the first therapeutic priority is to establish rapport and trust so that she will allow physical contact. The therapist begins a program of yoga and controlled breathing to improve Alyssa's ability to manage stress. As Alyssa develops trust in her therapist, she is more open to range of motion, weight bearing, mirror therapy, and progressive desensitization embedded within her yoga routines.

1. Why is yoga a good choice of therapeutic activity for this patient?
2. What biosocial concerns must be addressed along with those related to improving Alyssa's physical functioning?

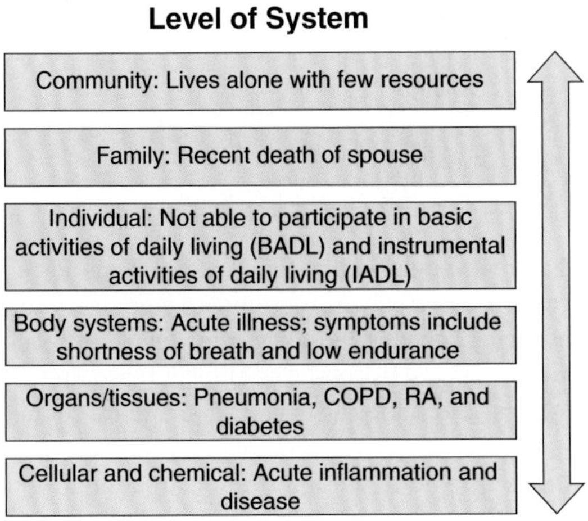

Level of System

Community: Lives alone with few resources
Family: Recent death of spouse
Individual: Not able to participate in basic activities of daily living (BADL) and instrumental activities of daily living (IADL)
Body systems: Acute illness; symptoms include shortness of breath and low endurance
Organs/tissues: Pneumonia, COPD, RA, and diabetes
Cellular and chemical: Acute inflammation and disease

Figure 5-3   Case 5-1: The occupational therapist working with Mary must create an intervention plan that addresses all levels of systems affected by her illness and personal situation. COPD, chronic obstructive pulmonary disease; RA, rheumatoid arthritis.

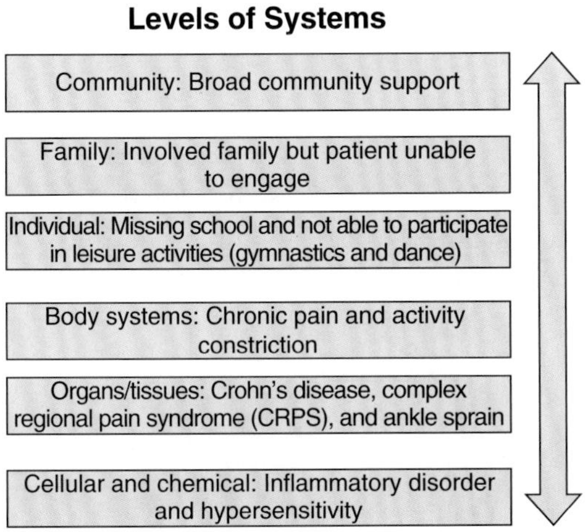

Levels of Systems

Community: Broad community support
Family: Involved family but patient unable to engage
Individual: Missing school and not able to participate in leisure activities (gymnastics and dance)
Body systems: Chronic pain and activity constriction
Organs/tissues: Crohn's disease, complex regional pain syndrome (CRPS), and ankle sprain
Cellular and chemical: Inflammatory disorder and hypersensitivity

Figure 5-4   Case 5-2: The occupational therapist working with Alyssa must create an intervention plan that addresses all levels of systems affected by her illness and personal situation.

 ## Contemporary Clinical Reasoning

Mary Reilly's NOBA method originated in the second half of the 20th century as a response to reductionism, and the approach was a reconnection to the profession's early fidelity to its core philosophy about occupation. As a framework for organizing and integrating clinical reasoning, it integrates occupational therapy's rich heritage and provides a useful point from which to consider intervention planning.

Hinojosa[15] pointed out a fragmentation that is present between factions of the contemporary occupational therapy profession. He identifies two competing science-based perspectives:

- Reductionistic (biomedical) models of practice
- Occupation-based interventions

Hinojosa argues that a singular view in favor of either perspective is harmful and states that pluralism is required because it does not promote polarization or fragmentation in the profession. This perspective is closely aligned to systems-level approaches and provides an updated framework for practice. His model of clinical reasoning states that the patient, practitioner, context, ethics, and scientific evidence are all essential components that must be considered in developing an intervention plan (Figure 5-5).

In the cases presented in the previous section, the occupational therapists used a systems methodology and a NOBA approach to develop action plans that involved

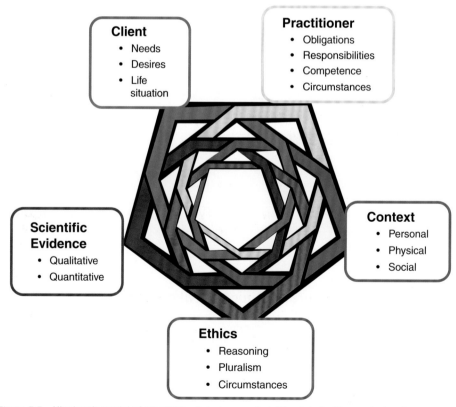

Figure 5-5   Hinojosa's model of pluralistic clinical reasoning. (Reprinted with permission from Hinojosa J. How society's philosophy has shaped occupational therapy practice for the past 100 years. *Open J Occup Ther.* 2017;5(2):1-12. doi:10.15453/2168-6408.1325.)

assessment and intervention at multiple levels of complexity. Both patients had biomedical and occupation-based concerns, and each situation required a unique method of problem solving to properly address the patient's concerns. Most importantly, if either therapist had attended to one concern over another, the patient's care would have been incomplete. Reilly's "magnificent purpose" (Reilly, 1962) is achieved by the unique ability of the occupational therapist to competently address concerns across levels.

Evaluating Approaches and Models of Practice

Occupational therapists are faced with fundamental questions in deciding how to best serve their patients/clients: "What do I do, and how do I know what is right and good?" These questions are easily answered when the therapist employs a sound rationale that is consistent with the traditions of the profession, the available evidence, and what is allowable under a legal scope of practice. The therapist must fully understand occupational therapy theory, evidence, and the laws regulating practice. "What should be done?" and "What is good?" are questions that can be answered from a perspective of pragmatism.

Pragmatism

Pragmatism is a philosophy promoted by William James in the late 19th century that has influenced the occupational therapy profession since its inception. At its core, pragmatism describes human behavior in terms of interacting systems of mind, body, and environment. William James was both philosopher and psychologist—he wanted his ideas to be applied.

Educator John Dewey expanded on James' ideas by promoting the concept that people learned by doing. Elwood Worcester, pastor of the Emmanuel Church in Boston also sanctioned this approach. Worcester stated, "I admired it [James' writings] so much that he was good enough to give it to me and permitted me to publish it in a series of tracts distributed by Emmanuel Church."[16(p239)]

These ideas were reflected in the early work of the Emmanuelists, of George Barton, in philosophical statements written by Adolph Meyer, and in the work of many other important contributors to the occupational therapy field, including Mary Reilly. Occupational therapists apply the concepts of pragmatism to their clinical reasoning through a series of steps that reflect the philosophy of doing, actual practice, and meeting commonsense needs.

The steps outlined in the following paragraphs incorporate the values of pragmatic clinical decision making. They reflect the philosophical core of the profession, the available scientific evidence, and the systemic realities that guide our encounters with patients/clients.

Step 1

Consider the person's need and understand that need from the perspective of occupation.

Therapists must avoid the pitfalls of eclecticism or reductionism by keeping occupation at the forefront of their thinking and begin their encounters with a deep understanding of the patient's need for occupation.

Step 2

Determine what evidence is available upon which a sound intervention plan can be based.

Evidence-based practice, as it is broadly defined, is the systematic methodology designed to integrate research evidence into the clinical reasoning process.[17] Concern has been raised about the application of a medical model of evidence-based practice to occupational therapy.[18] Although much evidence-based practice in medicine is based upon broad epidemiologic studies, the application to occupational therapy is more specific in that evidence-based practice should help clinicians "to make decisions about interventions that are effective for a specific client."[19(p131)] This approach of combining evidence-based practice with client-centeredness has been reported in the literature.[20]

Critical appraisal is an important component of evidence-based practice.[21(pp1-2)] Critical appraisal involves the analysis of data. Although evidence-based practice is an end, critical appraisal supplies a means. Tickle-Degnen[22] identified the steps that clinicians must take in integrating evidence into practice, but many clinicians are not fully participating in the process.[23,24]

Both patients/clients and reimbursement systems expect high-quality, effective, and efficient care. Appropriate clinical decision making is based on sound scientific data, and the therapist must interpret and apply the data in a meaningful, commonsense way to the individual's life experiences and specific needs.

Step 3

Understand the context and limitations.

The therapist must understand the context of where he or she is working and the limitations that are in place because of that context. Each locality may regulate occupational therapy practice, dictating the activities that can and cannot be done. Each work environment may also dictate the boundaries and scope of practice. The challenge is to understand and respect the patient's need for occupation, to identify the evidence that dictates best practice, and then to employ that thinking within the available space of the context.

Occupational therapy intervention for patients in an inpatient hospital unit will differ from that for patients in an outpatient facility. Likewise, intervention will differ for patients/clients who are in a private home versus those in a school or community setting. Each treatment context involves a different intervention plan based on policies and regulations that must be incorporated into clinical decision making.

Summary

- An eclectic approach to occupational therapy involves incorporating a variety of therapeutic principles and approaches to create the ideal treatment program for a specific patient/client. Although this approach may be appropriate in some situations, it may not be ideal for facilitating professional coherence and consistency of methodologies.

- Occupational therapists need to base their practice on sound theory to avoid decision making driven by limited, often environmental, contexts.

- Key principles of GST are that a system is made up of parts that interact to form a coherent whole and that complex systems share organizing principles. Systems are characterized by the dynamic interactions of their components, and those interactions can be complex and multidirectional.

- GST, embedded within the model of human occupation, provides a framework for inclusive thinking beyond reductionism. Occupational therapists need to focus at multiple levels of systems to understand an individual's occupational functioning.

- Clinical decision making can be influenced by environmental pressures such as institutional settings that use only standardized measures of patient/client status instead of considering the patient/client using a more expansive, holistic approach.

- The NOBA method states that clinicians should *not only* focus on biomedical or reductionistic science, *but also* attend to biosocial concerns. This approach emphasizes a focus on the range of impact throughout multiple systems.

- The two major influences on contemporary clinical reasoning are reductionistic (biomedical) models of practice and occupation-based interventions. A pluralistic approach integrates both of these influences.

- The patient/client, practitioner, context, ethics, and scientific evidence are essential components that must be considered in developing an intervention plan.

- Effective occupational therapy practice is based on careful and pragmatic balancing of the patient's occupational needs, the science supporting evidence-based practice, and contextual limitations and demands.

Reflect and Apply

Individual activity: Think about and record your answers to the following questions

1. Choose a health-related problem or diagnosis that you are familiar with and create a GST chart using the structure shown in Figures 5-3 and 5-4. Consider how the selected problem or diagnosis impacts systems at multiple levels.
2. Review the GST chart you created. Have you seen this problem being addressed by an occupational therapist? If so, what did you observe? In light of a systems perspective, would you suggest alternate methods of approaching the problem?

Small group discussion

1. Choose one GST chart and discuss how occupational therapy intervention planning might change based on
   - location of service delivery.
   - acute or chronic nature of the health concern.

- progression of the health concern.
- expertise of the therapist or access to resources.
- the available resources of the patient.
- any other factors you can consider.

Review Questions

1. An occupational therapist chooses to administer goniometric testing, a sensory test, and an ADL observation to a child who has cerebral palsy. This approach reflects the use of which approach or model?

    a. Eclectic approach
    b. Sensory processing model
    c. NOBA approach
    d. Biomechanical model

2. An occupational therapist is encouraged to use certain educationally relevant tests in a school setting. In this situation, practice is being dictated by

    a. therapist judgment.
    b. practice setting.
    c. evidence-based practice.
    d. unifying occupational therapy theory.

3. Which group of models can be most closely associated with a NOBA method?

    a. Sensory processing
    b. Cognitive disabilities
    c. Occupation-based
    d. Biomechanical

4. A GST approach is best for understanding

    a. muscle spindle excitation and impact on muscle tone.
    b. the insulin resistance of cells in prediabetes.
    c. the social policy for genetics counseling.
    d. the impact of osteoporosis on fracture healing.

5. The pressure to focus attention on elements of bed positioning, early mobility, and medical stability will be greatest for an occupational therapist working in which type of unit?

    a. General medical unit
    b. Intensive care unit
    c. Surgical step down unit
    d. Specialty cardiac unit

6. An occupational therapist working in a neonatal intensive care unit can use a NOBA approach by attending to which of the following concerns for a term baby admitted to the unit with severe birth asphyxia?

   a. Adhering to a low stimulation protocol during hypothermia protocol
   b. Encouraging the family to visit and bond with the infant
   c. Referral to the early intervention program
   d. All of the above

References

1. Wood W. Legitimizing occupational therapy's knowledge. *Am J Occup Ther*. 1996;50:626-634.
2. Shannon PD. The derailment of occupational therapy. *Am J Occup Ther*. 1977;31:229-234.
3. Ikiugu MN, Sames KM, Lauckner H. Use of theoretical conceptual practice models by occupational therapists in the US: a pilot survey. *Int J Ther Rehab*. 2012;19(11):629-639.
4. Ikiugu MN, Smallfield S, Condit C. A framework for combining theoretical conceptual practice models in occupational therapy practice. *Can J Occup Ther*. 2009;76(3):62-170.
5. Safran JD, Messer SB. Psychotherapy integration: a postmodern critique. *Clin Psychol*. 1997;4:140-152. doi:10.1111/j.1468-2850.1997.tb00106.x.
6. Reed KL, Sanderson SN. *Concepts of Occupational Therapy*. 4th ed. Philadelphia, PA: Lippincott Williams & Wilkins; 1999.
7. Wong SR, Fisher G. Comparing and using occupation-focused models. *Occup Ther Health Care*. 2015;29:297-315. doi:10.3109/07380577.2015.1010130.
8. Boniface G. Defining occupational therapy theory. In: Boniface G, Seymour A, eds. *Using Occupational Therapy Theory in Practice*. Gloucester, England: Wiley-Blackwell Company; 2012.
9. Kielhofner G, Burke JP. A model of human occupation, part 1. Conceptual framework and content. *Am J Occup Ther*. 1980;34:572-581.
10. Von Bertalanffy L. General systems theory: a critical review. In: Buckley W, ed. *Modern Systems Research for the Behavioral Scientist*. Chicago, IL: Aldine Press; 1968.
11. Boulding K. General systems theory: the skeleton of science. In: Buckley W, ed. *Modern Systems Research for the Behavioral Scientist*. Chicago, IL: Aldine Press; 1968.
12. Kielhofner G. General systems theory: implications for theory and action in occupational therapy. *Am J Occup Ther*. 1978;32:637-645.
13. Reilly M. Occupational therapy can be one of the great ideas of 20th century medicine. *Am J Occup Ther*. 1962;16:1-9.
14. Gutman SA, Mortera MH, Hinojosa J, Kramer P. Revision of the occupational therapy practice framework. *Am J Occup Ther*. 2007;61(1):119-126.
15. Hinojosa J. How society's philosophy has shaped occupational therapy practice for the past 100 years. *Open J Occup Ther*. 2017;5(2):1-12. doi:10.15453/2168-6408.1325.
16. Worcester E. *Body, Mind, and Spirit*. Boston, MA: Marshall Jones; 1931.
17. Tickle-Degnen L. Evidence based practice forum: organizing, evaluating, and using evidence in occupational therapy practice. *Am J Occup Ther*. 1999;53:537-539.
18. Canadian Association of Occupational Therapy. Joint position statement on evidence-based occupational therapy. *Can J Occup Ther*. 1999;66:267-273.
19. Law M, Baum C. Evidence-based occupational therapy. *Can J Occup Ther*. 1998;65:131-135.
20. Egan M, Dubouloz CJ, von Zweck C, Vallerand J. The client-centered evidence-based practice of occupational therapy. *Can J Occup Ther*. 1998;65:136-143.
21. Crombie IK. *The Pocket Guide to Critical Appraisal*. London, England: BMJ Publishing Group; 1996.

22. Tickle-Degnen L. Evidence-based practice forum: teaching evidence based practice. *Am J Occup Ther*. 2000;54:559-560.

23. Dysart AM, Tomlin GS. Factors related to evidence-based practice among U.S. occupational therapy clinicians. *Am J Occup Ther*. 2002;56:275-284.

24. Rappolt S, Tassone M. How rehabilitation therapists gather, evaluate, and implement new knowledge. *J Contin Edu Health Prof*. 2002;22;170-180.

6 The Biomechanical Model

Our body is not merely so many pounds of flesh and bone figuring as a machine, with an abstract mind or soul added to it. It is throughout a live organism pulsating with its rhythm of rest and activity, beating time (as we might say) in ever so many ways, most readily intelligible and in full bloom of its nature when it feels itself as one of those great self-guiding energy-transformers which constitute the real world of living beings.

—Adolph Meyer[1]
Archives of Occupational Therapy

Chapter Outline

Learning Objectives

1. Explain the origins of the biomechanical model.
2. Identify the key concepts and principles of the biomechanical model.
3. Describe how biomechanical principles are applied to various types of occupational therapy interventions.
4. Outline ways that biomechanical principles can be integrated into occupation-based models.

Key Terms

adaptation/compensation
biomechanical model
cardiovascular endurance
dynamometer
functional movement
goniometer
maintenance
muscular endurance
orthotic
postural control
posture
prevention
range of motion
remediation/rehabilitation
strength
work hardening

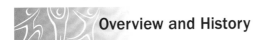 ## Overview and History

The **biomechanical model** is used in occupational therapy to address problems with **functional movement** (movement required to engage in daily occupations). Long-term care, hospital, and rehabilitation facilities are settings in which biomechanical interventions are commonly used. In clinical practice in physical disabilities settings, the biomechanical model is reported as the most commonly used practice model by entry-level occupational therapists.[2]

Occupational therapy practitioners use the biomechanical model in their work with many different patient populations. For example, a therapist in an early intervention setting might use principles of the biomechanical model when making range-of-motion (ROM) recommendations for a child who has torticollis (abnormal contraction of muscles of the neck). A practitioner in a school setting might make recommendations to improve sitting posture for a child with a neuromuscular disorder. A therapist in a behavioral setting for young adults might need to carry over an exercise and splinting program for a resident who fractured her hand.

The biomechanical model is also used in settings where it would be commonly expected, such as when teaching a hospital patient how to remove a brace to complete activities of daily living (ADL) after back surgery or in an acute rehabilitation facility helping a patient regain strength and mobility after fractures due to a motor vehicle crash. Occupational therapists in all settings use elements of the biomechanical model.

History of the Biomechanical Approach

Improving a person's physical movement has been a driving factor in occupational therapy since its inception. Recall that George Barton lost part of a foot to frostbite and suffered from partial paralysis. He established Consolation House in Clifton Springs, New York, in 1914 as a recuperative center for himself and others: "Paralyzed in his left side, he could scarcely do more than stand. With no motion possible in his left hand and arm, he used his own body as a clinic to work out the problem of rehabilitating himself."[3]

Shortly after conducting his experiments in physical reeducation, Barton began publishing articles describing the use of occupational therapy as a treatment for problems as simple as a child's broken bone to as complex as returning wounded soldiers to work.[4] Influenced by engineers Frank and Lillian Gilbreth and their ideas about efficiency, work flow, and motion studies, Barton applied the principles of biomechanical analysis to determine which occupations would be best to facilitate desired human movement.[5,6] Barton considered many of his observations to be commonsense analysis but also recognized that this work had never been submitted in the form of scientific proof and applied to what was then called reeducation (rehabilitation).

The biomechanical model was also based on the work of several other influential theoreticians and practitioners, including Bird Baldwin, Marjorie Taylor, and Sidney Licht.[7] Occupational therapists have expanded beyond the core biomechanical principles by pioneering efforts to document practice skills in the areas of splinting, physical agent modalities, and pain management.

In addition, interdisciplinary measurement and outcomes reporting in rehabilitation has been bolstered by the development of widely used assessment tools such as the Functional Independence Measure, a tool used to evaluate a patient's level of disability and change in status in response to rehabilitation or medical intervention.[8]

As identified by Stewart and Di Rezze[9] "very little contemporary occupational therapy literature is theoretical or conceptual about the physical determinants of occupation. Most of the current literature in this area is practical, applied, evidence-based, and not theoretical." Biomechanical and physical dysfunction principles applied in an occupational therapy context are documented in widely used comprehensive textbooks.[10,11]

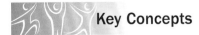

Key Concepts

The biomechanical model relies on an understanding of the basic physical principles of force and motion. This force and motion is analyzed using simple machine terms:

- Bones act as levers.
- Joints act as an axis around which movement occurs.
- Force is produced by muscles acting on bones and joints.

The biomechanical model focuses on general principles seen as critical for occupational functioning. These include ROM, strength, endurance, and postural control (Figure 6-1). Additional elements of balance, simple sensation, and pain perception are sometimes included in this model. These common elements are sometimes extended into simple performance of ADL, particularly mobility and self-care functions. The principles of inertia and acceleration are also important in the biomechanical model and are used to construct a basic understanding of movement problems.

Range of Motion

Range of motion (ROM) refers to the amount of movement possible at a joint. *Active range of motion* (AROM) is the amount of movement at a joint when the patient completes the movement on his/her own without assistance. *Passive range of motion* (PROM) is the amount of movement possible at a joint when the movement is performed with assistance from an outside force, such as the occupational therapist.

ROM is typically measured with a device known as a **goniometer** (Figure 6-2). It is critical for occupational therapists working with patients with restricted joint movement to become proficient in this measurement. Standardized procedures for conducting goniometric assessment are used to ensure the validity of the result.

Newer methods for assessing ROM using smart phone inclinometers are being developed, but their accuracy is still being assessed.[12,13] Methods used to improve a patient's

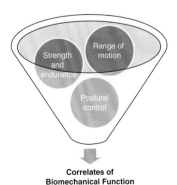

**Correlates of
Biomechanical Function**

Figure 6-1   Key concepts of the biomechanical model are range of motion, strength, endurance, and postural control.

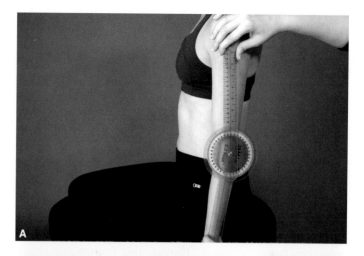

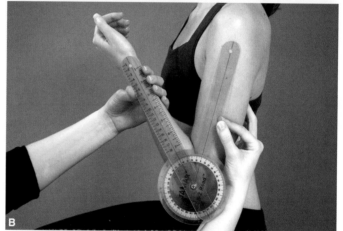

Figure 6-2   Goniometer being used to measure (A) elbow extension and (B) elbow flexion. (Reprinted with permission from Radomski MV, Latham CAT. *Occupational Therapy for Physical Dysfunction*. Philadelphia, PA: Wolters Kluwer Health | Lippincott Williams & Wilkins; 2014.)

ROM include passive movement by the therapist (PROM) and engaging the patient in exercise or activity under their own control (AROM). Therapists commonly grade movement experiences to meet individual patient needs.

Strength

Strength refers to the amount of available muscle power a person can activate. Strength is often measured using a standardized manual muscle test (MMT). In this kind of test, the patient moves his/her limb while opposing physical resistance is applied by the therapist. The patient's strength is assigned a numerical value based on the amount of resistance applied.

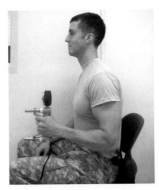

Figure 6-3   Dynamometer being used to measure grasp strength. (Reprinted with permission from Radomski MV, Latham CAT. *Occupational Therapy for Physical Dysfunction*. Philadelphia, PA: Wolters Kluwer Health | Lippincott Williams & Wilkins; 2014.)

Strength can also be measured using grip **dynamometers** (Figure 6-3) or other computerized devices that can precisely measure torque and muscle power. When using dynamometers, it is important for practitioners to carefully follow device instructions and to standardize administration so that results can be reliably interpreted.

Patients with muscle weakness may be guided to engage in strengthening activities to increase the muscles' ability to produce force. Various methodologies for strength training can be used, including isometric or concentric/eccentric muscle contractions. Therapists commonly grade strengthening exercises and activities to meet individual patient needs.

Endurance

Muscular endurance refers to the ability to sustain muscular activity over a specified period of time or to complete a specific task. **Cardiovascular endurance** refers to the ability of the circulatory and respiratory systems to deliver oxygenated blood to all body systems to meet metabolic demands. Occupational therapists commonly work with patients who have either or both kinds of endurance problems. In the context of occupational therapy, endurance may also be called *activity tolerance*.

Practitioners measure cardiovascular endurance by monitoring vital signs, including heart and respiratory rate, and how long it may take a patient to recover to a baseline following activity. The level of monitoring can be very sophisticated in the context of a cardiac rehabilitation unit, which is a specialty area of practice. More commonly, occupational therapy practitioners assess with simple cardiac or respiratory rate measurements. Therapists also use assessment tools such as the Borg Perceived Exertion Scale.[14] This assessment measures the patient's perception of how hard they are working.

Muscle endurance is measured as part of manual muscle testing. Alternately, functional observations of a patient completing ADL are also very helpful for determining muscular endurance to complete a task. More sophisticated and complex measurement of endurance can be done using computerized dynamometer systems such as the Baltimore therapeutic equipment or Biodex systems.

Therapists encounter many patients with endurance problems, particularly in acute care and long-term care settings where patients may be physically weak due to illness. Therapists grade exercise and activity to meet the endurance levels of their patients.

Postural Control

Posture is the position of the limbs or the carriage of the body as a whole. **Postural control**, which is closely related to balance, refers to a person's ability to maintain the center of gravity over his or her base of support. This ability is required to maintain a core stability that allows for controlled movement of the extremities through space. A carefully balanced and dynamic interplay of factors is required at different levels for the performance of different tasks. For example, different levels of ROM, strength, and endurance are required to sit at a desk versus those required to walk across a room. Limitations in strength, ROM, and endurance can all impact postural control, depending on task demands.

Interventions Using the Biomechanical Model

Depending on patient needs, interventions may include prevention, remediation/rehabilitation, adaptation/compensation, and maintenance of function (Figure 6-4 and Table 6-1). The studies cited in the following sections serve as examples of various types of evidence-based strategies, and there are many more examples in the literature that demonstrate how occupational therapists are using the biomechanical model in clinical practice.

Prevention

Prevention refers to an intervention strategy designed to avoid negative outcomes and to promote overall health and well-being. Many occupational therapists, especially those who work with elderly and disabled patients, are interested in strategies for the prevention of falls. Clemson et al[15] described their "lifestyle approach to reducing falls through exercise" as embedding balance and lower-limb strength training into daily routines. Their program was effective in reducing falls of at-risk participants. This type of program is a good example of prevention methodologies based on biomechanical principles that are commonly used in therapy.

Remediation/Rehabilitation

Remediation/rehabilitation refers to restoration of function through targeted training based on evidence-based assessment and intervention planning. Occupational therapists employ biomechanical remediation training for patients who are acutely ill or who are experiencing functional performance difficulties. For example, Valdes and von der Heyde[16] describe a review of evidence in support of a best-practice methodology for an exercise program for patients with arthritis in the carpometacarpal joint of the thumb.

Ma and Trombly[17] completed a kinematic analysis of a sequentially graded task and found that repeated movement increased force velocity and demand on motor efficiency. This study provided helpful support for the use of biomechanical task analysis and gradation of therapy tasks to improve motor skill in elderly patients. Remediation and rehabilitation methodologies are commonly employed in hospitals, long-term care facilities, home care, and many other settings.

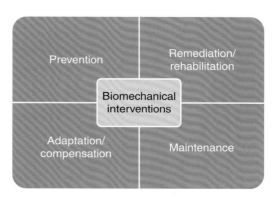

Figure 6-4   Biomechanical intervention strategies.

Table 6-1
Biomechanical Model

THEORY AND KEY READINGS	DEFINING FUNCTION	DEFINING DYSFUNCTION	ASSESSMENT	INTERVENTION
The biomechanical model has been used since the beginnings of the profession, evidenced by the work of Barton, Baldwin, Taylor, Licht, and many others.[5,30,31]	Having the requisite strength, range of motion, endurance, coordination, and other physical characteristics required for participation in occupations	Impairments in the structure and function of muscles, joints, bones, and associated structures so that movement is less efficient	• Goniometry • Manual muscle testing • Endurance testing • Fine and gross motor skills assessments • Postural assessment • Task analysis • Time and motion studies	• Use of physical agent modalities to improve physiologic conditions supporting movement • Orthotic or prosthetic training to support biomechanical function • Improving mobility through active or passive range of motion • Strengthening through progressive-resistive training and exercise • Improving functional activity tolerance through endurance training • Motor skills training • Use of any activity to achieve the above goals

Adaptation/Compensation

Adaptation/compensation refers to modifying a task (Figure 6-5) or environment to support occupational performance. For example, an occupational therapist may provide a long-handled reacher or dressing stick (Figure 6-6) to a patient recovering from spinal surgery. Because the patient is prevented from bending, a reacher or dressing stick can be used to assist with dressing tasks.

It is important for therapists to employ evidence-based principles when recommending adaptive equipment. Maitra et al[18] determined that the motor skills required for using a reacher were different than those used to reach and grasp normally. Their findings support the need to make sure that patients are given adequate training and practice opportunity to learn new motor skills needed for employing adaptive devices. Therapists must also involve patients in decision making about what type of adaptive equipment and training are most appropriate to improve therapy outcomes.[19]

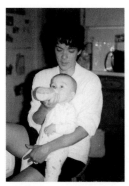

Figure 6-5   Woman with mild left hemiparesis using an alternate feeding position to give her baby a bottle. (Reprinted with permission from Radomski MV, Latham CAT. *Occupational Therapy for Physical Dysfunction*. Philadelphia, PA: Wolters Kluwer Health | Lippincott Williams & Wilkins; 2014.)

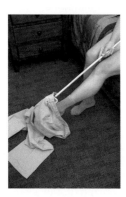

Figure 6-6   Woman using a dressing stick to assist with putting on clothes. (Reprinted with permission from Radomski MV, Latham CAT. *Occupational Therapy for Physical Dysfunction*. Philadelphia, PA: Wolters Kluwer Health | Lippincott Williams & Wilkins; 2014.)

Maintenance

Maintenance refers to interventions designed to maintain a certain level of skill or ability. Maintenance-level interventions for long-term care residents have received increased attention in the United States because of a 2013 court case that supported Medicare reimbursement for this therapy approach. The *Jimmo v. Sebelius* case determined that even if full recovery or patient improvement is not possible, Medicare may provide funding of skilled services to prevent further deterioration or to preserve current capabilities. An appropriately licensed therapist is required to plan and provide the intervention.

Maintenance-level interventions are not restricted to long-term care settings for adults. Another commonly employed methodology is the use of **orthotics** for children who have cerebral palsy. However, researchers are still investigating if there is enough evidence to support the use of orthotics for maintaining ROM and preventing joint contractures in patients who have cerebral palsy.[20]

Work Applications

Ergonomics and work hardening are practice contexts outside of the traditional medical model that are strongly associated with biomechanical principles. *Ergonomics* refers to the study of efficiency within a work environment. It is an area studied across the interdisciplinary professions of occupational therapy, industrial engineering, human factors engineering, psychology, management, and many others. Efficiency, as it relates to biomechanical principles, is an important concept because avoiding workplace injuries is an important goal in all employment settings.

Although many manual and repetitive assembly tasks are accomplished using automation and robotics, injuries from repetitive strain and poor workplace design and safety are still a significant problem. It is estimated that the annual cost of all workplace injuries in the United States is over $250 billion, a cost shared by all of society because only 25% of those costs are covered through the worker's compensation system.[21]

Occupational therapists use their knowledge of biomechanics to prevent injuries in the workplace and to help rehabilitate workers to enable their return to the work environment. An *ergonomic assessment* includes a thorough evaluation of an individual's workstation and associated analysis of job tasks, including the specific biomechanical elements required to complete all work activities. Recommendations are made for modifying the environment or the task to prevent or lessen the risk of occupational injury.

Work hardening refers to a systematized method of physical reconditioning that helps injured workers return to their employment. It is considered a phase of rehabilitation that occurs after the acute or medical phase. This type of programming is highly structured and individualized, with consideration given to the specific demands of the job as well as the physical capacity of the worker. The objective of work hardening is to restore physical and behavioral work habits so that the individual can safely and effectively resume employment.

Pain and the Biomechanical Model

Pain is a topic frequently framed within a biomechanical model because of the significant way that its presence can impact musculoskeletal function. Physical pain is often defined as being either nociceptive (originating from damage to body tissues) or neuropathic (originating from actual nerve damage). Pain is commonly treated with physician-prescribed and over-the-counter medications. Many occupational therapy approaches that arise out of the biomechanical model also follow this framework and suggest the use of physical agent modalities such as thermal and electrotherapeutic methods to reduce pain.

Peripheral and central nervous system processing may modify nociception, and behavioral/emotional states may also influence the perception of pain.[22] Chronic pain syndromes can often lead to long-term disability and loss of occupational functioning; for this reason, they have been studied extensively and are of interest to occupational therapy practitioners who describe their approach in biopsychosocial terms, extending their intervention beyond a biomechanical model.

Still, the understanding of pain is deeply rooted in reductionistic and physical terms, and the current problem of prescription drug overuse is an unfortunate result. As biopsychosocial framing has not successfully changed thinking, and as the societal cost of pain continues to be severe in both financial and human terms, some are calling for a new understanding of pain in sociopsychobiologic terms.[23] Expanding the understanding of pain beyond its strictly physical elements may help redirect intervention away from a singular reductionistic and biomechanical perspective. This idea represents a similar perspective to that seen in the NOBA methodology, respecting the reductionistic elements but remembering to understand the phenomenon in more broad systems terms.

Integrating Biomechanical Principles Into Occupation-Based Models

Occupational therapy clinicians state that their practice environments include constraints that make occupation-based intervention difficult. For example, Australian therapists report that workplace expectations for impairment-level practice hinder the application of occupation-based concepts into their interventions.[24] They also state that their university educators did not provide an integrated or consistent approach for helping them learn how to overcome these barriers. These issues may account for the primacy of biomechanical and reductionistic methodologies in clinical practice.

In addition, there will always be a certain amount of pressure from facilities to direct practice so that it will improve financial outcomes.[25,26] These pressures are often present in long-term care, hospital, and rehabilitation contexts where biomechanical interventions are commonly used.

Several authors have researched methods for integrating biomechanical and occupation-based approaches. A study comparing therapy based on an integrated intervention model with therapy based on a biomechanical rehabilitation model found no real differences in functional outcomes (recovery from hip fracture) among participants in both groups, but patients in the integrated model group reported higher overall satisfaction with their therapy and outcome.[27]

Case-based models of integrating occupation-based and biomechanical approaches have been described for patients with lateral epicondylitis[28] and for patients with post-surgical correction of joint deformity due to lupus-related arthritis.[29]

Occupational therapists need to be fluent in their ability to understand how to implement a NOBA methodology (see Chapter 5) to address both biomedical and biosocial patient needs and to advocate for best-practice strategies at their clinical worksites.

CASE 6-1 *Edward*

Edward is a 75-year-old man who cares for his wife who has a moderate degree of dementia. One night, his wife woke up, was confused, and began shouting. The noise startled the family dog, who bit Edward's right (nondominant) hand. The bite injury caused a flexor tendon rupture of the right third digit. He had a flexor tendon repair and was given a temporary splint. After 6 weeks, PROM was allowed. The therapist received a new order to begin gentle strengthening.

Motor and Sensory Skills

ROM is nearly within normal limits in protected positions, but there is passive insufficiency of the long finger flexors. He has mild edema and pain, particularly in the morning, but this resolves as the day progresses. Grip and pinch strength is severely limited. He can complete simple movements, and the doctor has just cleared him to begin resistive exercise. Edward reports that sensation is diminished throughout his palm and on the volar surfaces of digits II and III.

Summary of Biomechanical Dysfunction and Impact on Occupation

Edward is retired and has primary caregiving responsibility for his wife. He normally is responsible for all the home-management tasks as well as assisting his wife with bathing and dressing, and he was struggling with these tasks even before his injury. The assistance she requires can vary from supervision to moderate assistance. Because of pain and limitations from immobilization and splinting, he has not been able to complete these tasks and had to hire a home health aide and a housekeeping service on a temporary basis.

Edward has also been limited in completing his own personal care. Previously meticulous about his own appearance, he is upset about having to wear shirts and pants with no buttons (gym wear) and having to complete his hygiene at the bedside because he does not feel safe in the shower without the use of both hands. The home health aide has been helping him wash his hair twice a week, which is significantly below his usual preference.

Edward had to make the very difficult decision to surrender the family dog to a local humane society for a temporary foster placement. He was unable to care for the dog and fears another biting incident because current activity in the household can seem confusing to an animal.

In summary, Edward has a relatively uncomplicated flexor tendon injury in his nondominant hand, and his physical healing following this injury has been progressing to his surgeon's satisfaction. However, he is experiencing significant occupational dysfunction given the complex demands that this injury places on his ability to complete his usual occupations of husband, caregiver, and home manager. He requires both biomechanical and occupational treatment approaches to address the complexity of these needs.

Sample Goal From Intervention Plan

Edward will improve AROM for combined wrist and finger extension to a normal range for completing nonresistive home-management tasks.

Intervention Techniques and Equipment Used

Initiate gentle passive wrist and finger extension exercises. Following passive exercise, encourage gentle AROM within available range for nonresistive or very light resistive movements. Encourage folding laundry and reaching for lightweight dinnerware or glassware to put it away. Instruct Edward to elevate his hand slightly when resting and consider splinting as appropriate for night positioning.

Sequence of intervention:

1. Improve passive ROM.
2. Encourage gentle AROM.
3. Incorporate functional tasks and control pain/edema.

Analysis

The occupational therapist should conduct a full and careful interview to understand Edward's needs and work with him collaboratively to set appropriate goals and choose sensible accommodations while he heals from this injury.

General postsurgical movement protocols are dictated by many hand surgeons, and specific instructions will often be provided for individual patients. As the doctor is most closely aware of the flexor tendon repair and postsurgical healing, occupational therapists should follow the instructions closely as prescribed and carefully document and communicate observations and notes to the physician for collaborative intervention planning.

Biomechanical strategies of remediation, prevention, compensation, and maintenance are all applied by the occupational therapist as part of a comprehensive intervention plan. However, simply focusing on these biomechanical elements would not constitute complete or compassionate care for Edward. The complexity of his occupational needs must be considered and steps should be taken to facilitate a return to occupational roles as quickly as possible.

Using the theoretical foundations, concepts, and assumptions inherent in the biomechanical model:

1. Consider the critical nature of following the doctor's postsurgical therapy protocol and instructions. How does knowledge of the biomechanical model support safety and positive medical outcomes for Edward?
2. When being interviewed by the occupational therapist, Edward complained of significant pain. List as many reasons as you can that might be contributing to Edward's pain perceptions.
3. Imagine this exact same injury happening to Edward when he was 20 years younger and still working as an automobile mechanic. Identify all the elements in this case study that would be different and that would require an alternate intervention approach.
4. Describe the expected outcome of the occupational therapy intervention process.

Summary

- The biomechanical model is used to address problems with functional movement (movement required to engage in daily occupations). Biomechanical interventions are commonly used in long-term care, hospital, and rehabilitation facilities.

- Improving a person's physical movement has been a driving factor in occupational therapy since its inception.

- The biomechanical model focuses on general principles seen as critical for occupational functioning. These include ROM (the amount of movement possible at a joint), strength (the amount of available muscle power a person can activate), endurance (the ability to sustain muscular activity over a specified period of time or to complete a specific task), and postural control (a person's ability to maintain the center of gravity over his or her base of support).

- Additional elements of balance, simple sensation, and pain perception are sometimes included in this model.

- Interventions may include prevention (avoiding negative outcomes and promoting overall health and well-being), remediation/rehabilitation (restoration of function through targeted training based on assessment and intervention planning), adaptation/

compensation (modifying a task or environment to support occupational performance), and maintenance of function.

• Occupational therapists need to understand how to implement a NOBA methodology to address both biomedical and biosocial patient needs and to advocate for best-practice strategies.

Reflect and Apply

1. Reflect on occupational therapy interventions that you and your classmates have observed in different settings, including hospitals, outpatient facilities, and rehabilitation and long-term care facilities. Which types of interventions did you observe as being the most commonly used?
2. Consider the time and productivity demands on occupational therapists in many settings. How might a therapist integrate more occupation-based concepts into their intervention planning?
3. Conduct a literature review on a condition of your choice that is commonly seen by occupational therapists for which a biomechanical approach might be used. Does the research discuss biomechanical elements only, or does it also discuss impact on occupational performance? How might a therapist implement an integrated biomechanical and occupation-based model for the condition you researched? How would those interventions change in different treatment settings?

Review Questions

1. What can be done to help ensure reliability of grip strength testing?

   a. Complete multiple ROM measures.
   b. Use the same dynamometer each time.
   c. Complete rapid MMT measures.
   d. Compare with perceived exertion.

2. An occupational therapist designs a ROM program to be carried out by nurses in a long-term care facility. This program can be *best* described as

   a. remediation.
   b. adaptation.
   c. compensation.
   d. maintenance.

3. An occupational therapist creates an after-school activity program because of concerns that the children are not getting enough physical activity. This program can be best described as

   a. remediation.
   b. compensation.
   c. prevention.
   d. adaptation.

4. An occupational therapist at an acute rehabilitation facility works specifically with patients who have had recent hip and knee replacements. The kind of therapy provided is most likely

   a. remediation.
   b. prevention.
   c. maintenance.
   d. adaptation.

5. Which factor is frequently reported by occupational therapists as being a barrier to integrating occupation-based treatment with biomechanical interventions?

   a. Therapist disinterest in the model
   b. Patient disinterest in the model
   c. Productivity and reimbursement demands
   d. Insurance companies only reimburse exercise programs.

6. Which assessment is *most appropriate* for measuring exertion and fatigue in a patient who is recovering from an acute hospitalization?

   a. Borg scale
   b. Manual muscle test
   c. ROM test
   d. Functional Independence Measure

7. A grocery store worker is recovering from carpal tunnel surgery. She was experiencing severe pain and loss of function in her hands because of injury caused from repeated scanning of items at the checkout counter. Following her acute rehabilitation, what kind of program would be best for helping her return to work?

   a. Immobilization with splints
   b. Use of physical agent modalities to reduce pain
   c. Work hardening
   d. All of the above

8. Which of the following biomechanical interventions would be *most appropriate* for a patient who has an acute wrist fracture?

   a. ROM
   b. Strengthening
   c. Coordination training
   d. Splinting

9. Which of the following statements about pain management is *true*?

   a. Pharmaceuticals are not effective in managing pain.
   b. Reductionistic perspectives on pain may contribute to overuse of pharmaceuticals.
   c. Occupational therapists should avoid moving patients who are in pain.
   d. Physical agent modalities are not effective in managing pain.

References

1. Meyer A. The philosophy of occupational therapy. *Arch Occup Ther*. 1922;1:1-10.
2. Bent M, Crist P, Florey L, Strickland L. A practice analysis of occupational therapy and impact on certification examination. *OTJR*. 2005;25(3):105-118.
3. Barton I. Consolation house: fifty years ago. *Am J Occup Ther*. 1968;22:340-345.
4. Barton GE. Occupational therapy and the war. *Trained Nurse Hosp Rev*. 1916;57:9-10.
5. Barton GE. The movies and the microscope. *Trained Nurse Hosp Rev*. 1917;58:193-197.
6. Gilbreth FB, Gilbreth LM. The engineer, the cripple, and the new education. *Am Soc Mech Eng Trans*. 1918;39:1149-1170.
7. Reed KL. *Models of Practice in Occupational Therapy*. Baltimore, MD: Williams and Wilkins; 1984.
8. Keith RA, Granger CV, Hamilton BB, Sherwin FS. The functional independence measure: a new tool for rehabilitation. *Adv Clin Rehabil*. 1987;1:6-18.
9. Stewart D, Di Rezze B. Occupational conceptual models associated with the physical determinants of occupation. In: McColl MA, Law MC, Stewart D, eds. *Theoretical Basis of Occupational Therapy*. 3rd ed. Thorofare, NJ: Slack Inc; 2015:95.
10. Pendleton HM, Schultz-Krohn W. *Pedretti's Occupational Therapy: Practice Skills for Physical Dysfunction*. St. Louis, MO: Elsevier; 2018.
11. Radomski MV, Latham CAT. *Occupational Therapy for Physical Dysfunction*. 7th ed. Baltimore, MD: Wolters Kluwer; 2014.
12. Jones A, Sealey R, Crowe M, Gordon S. Concurrent validity and reliability of the Simple Goniometer iPhone app compared with the Universal Goniometer. *Physiother Theory Prac*. 2014;30(7):512-516. doi:10.3109/09593985.2014.900835.
13. Mitchell K, Gutierrez SB, Sutton S, Morton S, Morgenthaler A. Reliability and validity of goniometric iPhone applications for the assessment of active shoulder external rotation. *Physiother Theory Pract*. 2014;30(7):521-525. doi:10.3109/09593985.2014.900593.
14. Borg G. *An introduction to Borg's RPE Scale*. Ithaca, NY: Movement Publications; 1985.
15. Clemson L, Singh MF, Bundy A, et al. LiFE Pilot Study: a randomised trial of balance and strength training embedded in daily life activity to reduce falls in older adults. *Australian Occup Ther J*. 2010;57(1):42-50. doi:10.1111/j.1440-1630.2009.00848.x.

16. Valdes K, von der Heyde R. An exercise program for carpometacarpal osteoarthritis based on bio-mechanical principles. *J Hand Ther*. 2012;25(3):251-263. doi:10.1016/j.jht.2012.03.008.

17. Ma H, Trombly CA. Effects of task complexity on reaction time and movement kinematics in elderly people. *Am J Occup Ther*. 2004;58(2):150-158.

18. Maitra KK, Philips K, Rice MS. Grasping naturally versus grasping with a reacher in people without disability: motor control and muscle activation differences. *Am J Occup Ther*. 2010;64(1):95-104.

19. Thomas WN, Pinkelman LA, Gardine CJ. The reasons for noncompliance with adaptive equipment in patients returning home after a total hip replacement. *Phys Occup Ther Geriatr*. 2010;28(2);170-180. doi:10.3109/02703181003698593.

20. Morris C, Bowers R, Ross K, Stevens P, Phillips D. Orthotic management of cerebral palsy: recommendations from a consensus conference. *NeuroRehabilitation*. 2011;28(1):37-46. doi:10.3233/NRE-2011-0630.

21. Leigh JP. Economic burden of occupational injury and illness in the United States. *Milbank Q*. 2011;89(4):728-772. doi:10.1111/j.1468-0009.2011.00648.x.

22. Melzack R, Wall P. Pain mechanisms: a new theory. *Science*. 1965;150:171-179.

23. Carr DB, Bradshaw YS. Time to flip the pain curriculum? *Anesthesiology*. 2014;120(1):12-14. doi:10.1097/ALN.0000000000000054.

24. Di Tommaso A, Isbel S, Scarvell J, Wicks A. Occupational therapists' perceptions of occupation in practice: an exploratory study. *Australian Occup Ther J*. 2016;63(3):206-213. doi:10.1111/1440-1630.12289.

25. Roberts PS, Robinson MR. Occupational therapy's role in preventing acute readmissions. *Am J Occup Ther*. 2014;8(3):254-259. doi:10.5014/ajot.2014.683001.

26. Rogers AT, Bai G, Lavin RA, Anderson GF. Higher hospital spending on occupational therapy is associated with lower readmission rates. *Med Care Res Rev*. 2017;74(6):668-686. doi:10.1177/1077558716666981.

27. Jackson J, Schkade J. Occupational adaptation model versus biomechanical-rehabilitation model in the treatment of patients with hip fractures. *Am J Occup Ther*. 2001;55(5):531-537.

28. Bachman S. Evidence-based approach to treating lateral epicondylitis using the occupational adaptation model. *Am J Occup Ther*. 2016;70(2):1-5. doi:10.5014/ajot.2016.016972.

29. Jack J, Estes RI. Documenting progress: hand therapy treatment shift from biomechanical to occupational adaptation. *Am J Occup Ther*. 2010;64(1):82-87.

30. Swaim LT, Taylor M. Occupational therapy for the orthopedic patient crippled by chronic disease. *Phys Med Rehabil*. 1925;4(3):171-176.

31. Licht S. Kinetic occupational therapy. In: Dunton WR, Licht S, eds. *Occupational Therapy: Principles and Practice*. Springfield, IL: Charles C Thomas; 1957:55-83.

When the sensory integrative capacity of the brain is sufficient to meet the demands of the environment, the child's response is efficient, creative, and satisfying. When the child experiences challenges to which he can respond effectively, he "has fun." To some extent, "fun" is the child's word for sensory integration.

—A. Jean Ayres[1]
Sensory Integration and the Child

Chapter Outline

Learning Objectives

1. Explain the origins of the sensory integration (SI) model.
2. Identify the key concepts and principles of the SI model.
3. Describe how the SI model has developed over time.
4. Outline ways that SI principles can be integrated into occupation-based models.

Key Terms

adaptive responses
fidelity
neuroplasticity
praxis

proprioception
sensory integration
sensory integration model
tactile
vestibular sense

Overview

The **sensory integration (SI) model** is an iconic approach in the occupational therapy profession, despite some uncertainty regarding definitions, classifications, and assumptions over the years. The SI model was introduced by Ayres.[1,2] As originally described by Ayres,[3(p5)] **sensory integration** is "the organization of sensation for use" (Figure 7-1). Sensory integration therapy (SIT) is most commonly used with children who have difficulties processing sensory information, but this approach has sometimes been applied to other populations. Ayres asserted that SI was an evolving concept, saying that "truth, like infinity, is to be forever approached but never reached."[2(p4)] This is evident in the continual revision and expansion of the original theory.

Although there have been changes to the original model, some elements have been very consistent over time. For example, the SI model relies on the concept of **neuroplasticity**, which is the brain's ability to form and reorganize synaptic connections in response to experience. Additional elements have been consistently included in descriptions of the SI model since its inception.

Original SI Concepts

Ayres' initial 1972 publication was a technical exploration of the model. In 1979, she published *Sensory Integration and the Child*, a book designed to educate parents and families. In 1989, she defined SI as the organization of sensations that make it possible to use the body effectively in the environment.[3(p11)] She believed that lack of SI was the cause of certain learning and developmental difficulties in children. Her goal was to create a model to guide occupational therapists in creating environments that would elicit adaptive responses that organize a child's brain, specifically in children who cannot do this on their own through typical play (Table 7-1).

Ayres' ideas focused on improving function of the *neocortex* (dorsal region of the cerebral cortex, Figure 7-2) by achieving integration at lower levels in the *neuraxis* (spinal cord, rhombencephalon, mesencephalon, and diencephalon, Figure 7-3). She often compared with this approach to the cortically directed perceptual-motor approaches.

Praxis is a cortically driven neurologic process by which people plan and direct motor action (planning a movement and then executing it). Ayres was interested in praxis

Table 7-1
Sensory Integration Model

THEORY AND KEY READINGS	DEFINING FUNCTION	DEFINING DYSFUNCTION	ASSESSMENT	INTERVENTION
The sensory integration model was introduced by A. Jean Ayres and has evolved since the 1970s.[1,2,18]	When people are able to organize sensation from their body and from the environment, which allows them to use their body effectively in the environment.	Deficits in processing and integrating sensory inputs interfere with conceptual and motor learning. Difficulties in planning and producing adaptive responses interfere with conceptual and motor learning. Atypical modulation of sensory inputs interferes with conceptual and motor learning.	• Sensory Integration and Praxis Tests[3] • Sensory Profile(s)[21] • Sensory Processing Measure[14] • Structured observations	• Ayres Sensory Integration, sometimes referred to as "classical" sensory integration therapy. Use of this model implies fidelity to structural and processing elements. • Intervention includes the therapist setting up the "just-right challenge" in the context of collaborative play, which will promote the child's development of adaptive responses. • Other researchers and practitioners do not adhere to fidelity measures and promote compensatory skill development, group therapy programs, passively applied sensory stimulation, and other alternative and complementary interventions.

because it relies on underlying SI that is difficult to measure. The end product of SI can be more easily measured by observing the actions of children engaged in play and other occupations. Ayres hypothesized that occupational therapy practitioners could make inferences about the underlying neurologic process of SI by observing the skilled actions of children. This led to her developing the Southern California Sensory Integration Tests and later the Sensory Integration and Praxis Tests.

SI interventions involve the use of activities designed to strengthen the individual's ability to register and integrate **tactile** inputs (sense of touch), balance, and **proprioception** (sense of where body parts are in space).

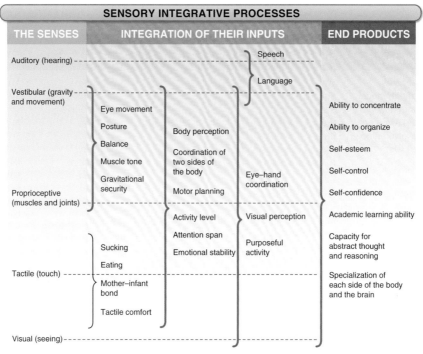

Figure 7-1   Ayres' chart outlining sensory integration processes. (Reprinted with permission from Boyt Schell BA, Gillen G, Scaffa ME, et al. *Willard and Spackman's Occupational Therapy.* 12th ed. Philadelphia, PA: Lippincott Williams & Wilkins/Wolters Kluwer; 2013.)

Vestibular sense is a complex sense related to the perception of body position, head orientation, posture, and motion. The vestibular system consists of structures of the inner

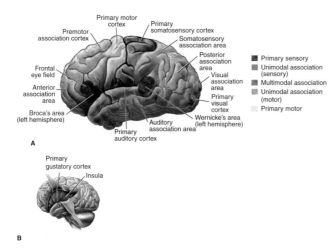

Figure 7-2   Functional areas of the cerebrum. A, Functional areas. B, The gustatory cortex and insula. (Reprinted with permission from McConnell TH, Hull KL. *Human Form, Human Function: Essentials of Anatomy & Physiology.* Baltimore, MD: Lippincott Williams & Wilkins; 2010.)

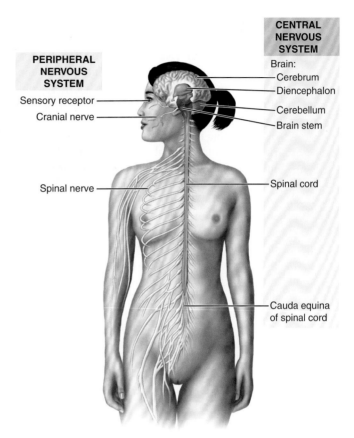

CENTRAL NERVOUS SYSTEM

Brain:
Cerebrum
Diencephalon
Cerebellum
Brain stem

PERIPHERAL NERVOUS SYSTEM

Sensory receptor
Cranial nerve

Spinal nerve

Spinal cord

Cauda equina of spinal cord

Figure 7-3   The central and peripheral nervous systems. (Reprinted with permission from McConnell TH, Hull KL. *Human Form, Human Function: Essentials of Anatomy & Physiology*. Baltimore, MD: Lippincott Williams & Wilkins; 2010.)

ear that send information to the brain about the location of the head in space. Vestibular information is predominantly processed in the brainstem. Proprioceptive and tactile processing is predominantly processed throughout the midbrain. According to Ayres, effective integration of these lower-brain systems would lead to **adaptive responses**, which are defined as successful, goal-directed actions that meet environmental demands.

SI was often expressed in terms of nervous system hierarchy, even though Ayres recognized that the brain functions as a whole.[2(p13)] Because of this preference, SI theory has historically focused more on tactile, proprioceptive, and vestibular sensory processing in lower-brain centers than on visual or auditory sensory processing in higher-brain centers.

Evolving SI Concepts

Su and Parham[4] completed a study to evaluate the validity of sensory system measures as distinct constructs. Specifically, the authors stated that one of their primary interests was to "test the discreteness of sensory system measures in preparation for further research examining whether functions of the tactile, vestibular, and proprioceptive systems serve as a foundation for visual and auditory functioning, as Ayres theory proposes." They found that there was a distinct statistical model that supported tactile, vestibular-proprioceptive, auditory, and visual functions, but that these could not be specifically linked to unidirectional models of hyper or hyper- or hyporesponsiveness.

These findings follow many other classification attempts that highlight the challenges of attempting to clarify the nature of sensory problems[5-9] (Tables 7-2 and 7-3). The categorization of foundational sensory systems that support vision and hearing in a hierarchical manner remains unclear, and lack of clarity in basic concepts is problematic for theory development and for designing evidence-based intervention plans.

This lack of fundamental clarity has plagued the SI model since its inception. Although some researchers focus on sensory systems, others focus on patterns of behavior associated with those systems. Some clinicians use passive sensory strategies such as swinging a child in a swing or applying tactile input to the extremities. In these examples, the therapist provides sensory input to a passive child. Others insist that all intervention must be "child directed" and must include the active engagement of the child. These differences in approach have been problematic because they contributed to a lack of consensus among SI practitioners and researchers.

Disagreement about terminology and naming conventions[10,11] and tepid acceptance from mainstream medical practitioners[12] have contributed to confusion around this model. The American Academy of Pediatrics (AAP) found it difficult to evaluate the effectiveness of SI therapy because of ". . . the wide spectrum of symptom severity and presentation, lack of consistent outcome measures, and family factors, which make response to therapy variable" (p. 1187).

Because of uncertainty surrounding this approach, the AAP suggests that parents review progress regularly when children receive these services. So, although this model

TABLE 7-2
Patterns of Sensory Integration Dysfunction Based on Ayres Sensory Integration

SENSORY INTEGRATION DYSFUNCTION	DESCRIPTION
Poor sensory perception	Difficulty in identifying, discriminating, and interpreting sensory information
Somatodyspraxia	Difficulty with motor planning based on processing somatosensory inputs
Vestibular and bilateral integration deficits	Inefficient vestibular processing and poor bilateral, postural, ocular, and sequencing functions
Visuodyspraxia	Difficulty with visual perception and visual motor skills

These descriptions have been validated in cluster and factor analytic studies.

Source: Ayres AJ. *The Sensory Integration and Praxis Tests*. Los Angeles, CA: Western Psychological Services; 1989; Mailloux Z, Mulligan S, Smith Roley S, et al. Verification and clarification of patterns of sensory integrative dysfunction. *Am J Occup Ther*. 2011;65:143-151; Mulligan S. Patterns of sensory integration dysfunction: a confirmatory factor analysis. *Am J Occup Ther*. 1998;52:819-828; and Mulligan S. Cluster analysis of scores of children on the sensory integration and praxis tests. *Occup Ther J Res*. 2000;20(4):256-270.

TABLE 7-3
Patterns of Sensory Reactivity Based on Ayres Sensory Integration

PATTERN	DESCRIPTION
Hyperreactivity to sensory input	Hypersensitivity or overresponsiveness to sensory inputs that interfere with participation
Hyporeactivity to sensory input	Hyposensitivity or underresponsiveness to sensory inputs that interfere with participation

These descriptions have been validated in cluster and factor analytic studies.

Source: Dunn W, Brown C. Factor analysis on the Sensory Profile from a national sample of children without disabilities. *Am J Occup Ther.* 1997;51:490-495, discussion 496-499; Dunn W. *Sensory Profile 2 User's Manual.* Bloomington, IN: Pearson; 2014; and Parham L, Ecker C, Miller-Kuhanek H, et al. *Sensory Processing Measure Manual.* Los Angeles, CA: Western Psychological Services; 2007.

has been widely discussed, researched, and adopted in various ways by occupational therapy practitioners, it still engenders a lot of controversy within and outside the profession.

Fidelity Measure for the SI Model

The term *fidelity* in a general sense means faithfulness to a person, cause, or belief. In occupational therapy research and practice, **fidelity** refers to the degree to which an intervention is implemented according to its underlying theoretical principles and procedural guidelines. Parham et al.[13,15] identified the core elements of Ayres Sensory Integration (ASI) and developed the ASI Fidelity Measure. They identified the structural and process elements of intervention that should be adhered to by researchers and clinicians (Figure 7-4). Adherence to these elements is believed to contribute to consistency of delivery that can improve clinical practice and research efforts.

Although the ASI Fidelity Measure is available, many studies report on sensory-based interventions that do not meet the criteria as measures of SI.[16] Often, therapists and researchers state that they are using a SI model but do not adhere to the identified structural and process elements. In Watling and Hauer's[16] review of studies that did adhere to those elements, there is initial evidence that SI intervention may be helpful for achieving family-stated goals. There was not good evidence for other sensory-based interventions such as the use of weighted products or implementation of auditory integration training.

Incorporating SI Into Occupation-Based Models

Many scholars have integrated SI theory into occupation-based intervention approaches by re-examining ways to broaden Ayres' original concepts. The integration of these two

SENSORY INTEGRATION MODEL	
STRUCTURAL ELEMENTS	**PROCESS ELEMENTS**
• Formal education of interveners • Professional background of interveners • Postprofessional SI training of interveners • SIPT or SCSIT certification • Clinical experience of interveners • Type of therapeutic equipment • Room setup • Supervision of interveners	• Arranges room to entice engagement • Creates a play context • Presents sensory opportunities • Presents challenges to elicit adaptive responses • Supports child's self-organization of behavior • Collaborates with child in activity choices • Helps child maintain optimal arousal • Maximizes child's experience of success • Ensures child's safety

Figure 7-4   Structural and process elements of Ayres Sensory Integration. SI, sensory integration; SCSIT, Southern California Sensory Integration Tests; SIPT, Sensory Integration and Praxis Tests.

models has been explored and documented for many years.[17,18(pxvii)] Although Ayres may not have explicitly described the impact that disordered sensory systems have on occupations, these concepts can be applied to develop a richer understanding of what it means to have sensory processing difficulties.

Florey[19] provided a useful framework for operationalizing a NOBA (not only but also) methodology in a pediatric context, although she was not specifically referring to a SI model. She identified several important types of knowledge that were needed when approaching a pediatric clinical problem:

* *Knowledge about pathology and disease.* The SI model provides rich opportunity to understand neurologic correlates of occupational behavior.
* *Understanding of growth and development*, which is key in both SI and occupation-based models.
* *Knowledge about play*, another area with strong points of commonality between models.
* *Knowledge of general systems theory.* Florey suggested that therapists need to apply their perspectives with a knowledge of open systems and the rules of hierarchy.

Relevant assessment tools might include play histories and observations and would also include consideration of self-care and school performance. Many of the core intervention constructs of the SI model are directly related to elements that reinforce exploratory, competency, and achievement behaviors of children (Figure 7-5).

Figure 7-6 outlines play-based intervention elements that make SI and occupation-based models compatible when used together within a NOBA orientation. Integration of the SI model into the occupational context of school-based practice has also been extensively described.[20] In any practice setting, the challenge to the therapist is to be aware of the fidelity issue and to maintain close adherence to structural and process elements when documenting and reporting use of the SI model.

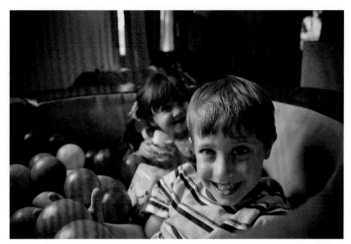

Figure 7-5   Playing in a ball pool provides tactile stimulation and resistance to movement, increasing the child's body awareness. (Courtesy of ABC Therapeutics.)

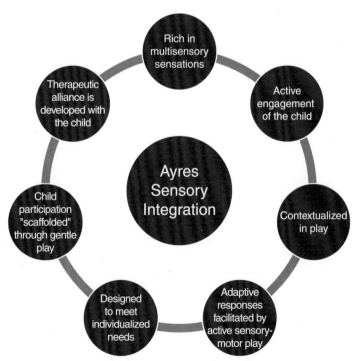

Figure 7-6   Play-based intervention elements that incorporate sensory integration into occupation-based models. (Adapted from Schaaf RC, Mailloux Z. *Clinician's Guide for Implementing Ayres Sensory Integration: Promoting Participation for Children With Autism*. Bethesda, MD: AOTA Press; 2015.)

Guidelines for Practice

Clinicians interested in using the SI model should follow these guidelines:

- Study the most up-to-date interpretations of concepts and assumptions from SI researchers. Evaluate research on the basis of studies that have maintained some fidelity to a standardized set of intervention protocols.
- Be careful to discern which interventions represent actual SI, as opposed to single modality sensory-based interventions, for which there has not been very good research evidence.
- Incorporate SI concepts into a broader understanding of childhood occupations such as play, self-care, and learning. On the basis of a long history, this aspect of the SI model may be one of its most important strengths.

CASE 7-1   *Luis*

Luis is a 5-year-old who recently started kindergarten at his local public elementary school. He is diagnosed with diabetes insipidus and growth hormone insufficiency, and his most recent occupational therapy evaluation occurred approximately 1½ years ago. He has been receiving occupation therapy services twice a week since that time. He also receives physical therapy, speech therapy, and special education services through the school district. His parents requested a private occupational therapy evaluation to document his current level of ability.

Luis was born via planned cesarean section due to breech positioning. He received supplemental oxygen at birth and had apnea and bradycardia monitors. Because of complications associated with his medical condition, he was previously very overweight, but he has lost 40 lb in the last year. His current weight is 64 lb. Developmental milestones have all been delayed. He had a brief stay of inpatient rehabilitation to stabilize his diet and develop a nutritional plan. Luis receives growth hormone injections and is followed by an endocrinologist. He is medicated with levothyroxine (Synthroid) and desmopressin (DDAVP).

Motor Behavior

Range of motion (ROM) is within normal limits. Luis has moderate hypotonia. He demonstrates delayed/slow equilibrium and protective responses from all positions. His posture is within functional limits; however, reduced strength causes postural kyphosis in sitting. He slouches over his work and keeps his face very close to the page. He has fair strength. Luis is not able to assume/maintain antigravity positions of prone extension or supine flexion, and he lacks power for sustained cocontraction. He has an emerging left-hand dominance. On a standardized test of motor skills, he scored between the 2nd and 5th percentiles in all areas.

Sensory Skills

Tactile system: Parent does not express any concerns about Luis's tactile skills.
Vestibular-proprioceptive system: Parent reports that Luis seems excessively fearful of movement, that he becomes easily upset when placed on riding or moving equipment, and that he has poor balance and is generally weak. Luis is weak and unsure of how to coordinate body movements. Parent stated that his grasp was so weak on a pencil that it makes his writing essentially nonfunctional.
Visual system: Parent reports that Luis has difficulty with letter identification and difficulty with other basic visual discrimination tasks. He can identify only a few letters in his name and scores below the 1st percentile on a standardized test of visual perceptual skills.

Summary of Sensory Dysfunction and Impact on Occupation

Luis demonstrates focal sensory difficulties in the areas of vestibular-proprioceptive processing and visual perception. It is likely that his severely overweight condition previously hindered his sensory-motor development. Because of extreme weight instability and lack of adequate motor play/experience, his praxis and motor development has been negatively impacted.

Visual perception difficulties are also notable and may be related to an inadequate sensory foundation for processing vestibular and proprioceptive information. Lack of typical movement experiences may also have a negative impact on the development of visual perceptual skills.

Functionally, Luis requires significant assistance for completing basic self-care routines including dressing and hygiene. He has difficulty with the motor skills needed to complete these tasks. He is able to feed himself using utensils.

Regarding academic skill development, Luis is interested in coloring and simple puzzles but demonstrates very little skill in this area. He can mark a page and can grossly imitate vertical and horizontal strokes. When attempting to copy a circle, he will resort to circular scribbling. He can snip with scissors but cannot cut on a line. He uses trial-and-error problem-solving to complete simple puzzles. Luis has difficulty with counting and inconsistently recognizes a few letters of the alphabet.

Overall play development is severely constricted. According to parental report and clinical observations, Luis engages in simple constructive and emerging fantasy play. He interacts better with adults than with his peers. Motor skill deficits limit his repertoire of play behaviors.

In summary, Luis's area of greatest difficulty is in poor vestibular-proprioceptive processing which causes delays in his motor skills. In particular, Luis's balance, locomotion, and motor coordination for functional navigation of his environment and gross motor play are most problematic. Fine motor skills for cutting and writing are also a significant need and are similarly impacted by poor sensory processing. Occupational functioning is challenged in all areas.
Sample goal from intervention plan: Luis will maintain balance on uneven surfaces while walking in/around school, 80% of trials.

Intervention Techniques/Equipment Used

Encourage parents to provide opportunities for safe gross motor play in the home and have Luis participate in play activities in the clinic. Grade the playing surface by encouraging play on trampoline (sitting) and progressing to equilibrium board and linear glider with feet on ground. Also, encourage play activities inside ball pit for combined surface instability and deep pressure stimulation. Alternatively, allow Luis to play in/around suspended equipment, allowing him to place toys on a moving surface while he is stable. Incorporate preferred fantasy play themes and grade by beginning with familiar play experiences.

Sequence of intervention:

1. Reduce hypersensitivity to movement.
2. Introduce linear vestibular stimulation. Use deep pressure as a modulator as needed.
3. Initiate simple balance activities, close to floor/feet on ground, with linear challenges.

Analysis

Luis has low muscle tone combined with gravitational insecurity. This combination of clinical signs indicates deficits in tonic processing of vestibular inputs within the brainstem most likely associated with impaired body scheme. Graded introduction to linear movement experiences combined with inhibitory inputs may help Luis tolerate the new movement experiences and improve posture and motor skill for learning and play.

Use the theoretical foundations, concepts, and assumptions inherent in the SI model to complete the following learning activities:

1. Reflecting on the concept of neuroplasticity, explain why providing opportunities for movement experiences is important during Luis's occupational therapy sessions.
2. Focusing on the idea of developing a therapeutic alliance with the child, list five different strategies that a practitioner might use to encourage sensory-based play for a child who does not prefer those experiences.
3. Review the case study and write a goal for Luis related to improving pencil control for writing in a school environment. Include a hypothesis of why the problem is happening, a sequence of suggested intervention activities, and rationale for your choices.
4. Describe the expected outcomes of the occupational therapy intervention process using an SI approach.

Summary

- The SI model was introduced by A. Jean Ayres, who described SI as "the organization of sensation for use."

- Ayres' ideas focused on improving function of the neocortex by achieving integration at lower levels in the neuraxis. SI theory focuses more on tactile, proprioceptive, and vestibular sensory processing than on visual or auditory sensory processing.

- SIT is used with people who have movement disorders and those with sensory processing problems. Interventions involve activities designed to strengthen the registration and integration of the individual's sense of touch, balance, and proprioception.

- Many of the core intervention constructs of the SI model are directly related to elements that reinforce exploratory, competency, and achievement behaviors of children.

- The ASI Fidelity Measure identifies the structural and process elements of intervention that should be adhered to for consistency in practice and for meaningful research.

- SI concepts should be applied along with a broader understanding of childhood occupations such as play, self-care, and learning.

Reflect and Apply

1. Reflect on therapy interactions you observed in pediatric settings. Did the therapists state they were employing an SI model? List structural and process elements that you observed that might support or refute that designation.
2. Working with a partner, complete a database search of SI research and identify three different articles. Assess the research as it relates to fidelity to relevant structural and process elements. Compare your results and see if there is evidence of increased fidelity in recent years.
3. More than any other concept in occupational therapy, the ideas about SI are accepted and used by other disciplines, parents, and the public in general. Conduct an online search and read about how widespread this model is. Do you think that this broad use of SI concepts has helped or hindered theory development? Explain your conclusions.

Review Questions

1. The concept of "fidelity" became important in the occupational therapy literature related to assessing the quality of research for which type of approach?

   a. Motor learning
   b. Sensory integration
   c. Biomechanical
   d. Perceptual motor

2. Sensory integration is best defined as

   a. a neurologic process that organizes sensory information from the environment.
   b. a neurologic process that organizes sensory information from one's own body.
   c. the ability to organize sensory information for use.
   d. the ability to process hierarchically complex information.

3. According to the AAP, what is important for doctors to communicate to their patients regarding sensory integration treatment programs?

   a. There is enough evidence to support sensory integration therapies.
   b. Sensory integration disorders have a 5% to 20% prevalence rate.
   c. Children generally require at least 6 months of sensory integration therapy.
   d. Parents should review progress regularly when children receive these services.

4. Which of the following treatment programs incorporates specific structural and process elements to ensure conceptual fidelity?

   a. Wilbarger Deep Pressure protocol
   b. The Ready approach
   c. The Alert program
   d. Ayres SI approach

5. Which of the following represent structural elements that should be present for an intervention to be properly defined as sensory integration?

   a. Sensory Integration and Praxis Tests certification
   b. Creating a play context
   c. Helping a child maintain optimal arousal
   d. Ensuring safety in the clinic environment

6. Which element was *not* identified by Florey as critical for occupation-based treatment planning in pediatrics?

   a. Being knowledgeable about pathology or disease
   b. Understanding the process of growth and development
   c. Advanced postprofessional training
   d. Being knowledgeable about play development

7. Ayres stated that the primary goal in sensory integration intervention is to

   a. improve postural-ocular responses for praxis.
   b. elicit adaptive responses that organize the child's brain.
   c. facilitate midline crossing and integration of primitive reflexes.
   d. discriminate tactile and proprioceptive contributions toward neurologic processing of sensory inputs.

8. The brain's ability to form and reorganize synaptic connections in response to experience is defined as

   a. classical conditioning.
   b. learning theory.
   c. proprioceptive learning.
   d. neuroplasticity.

References

1. Ayres AJ. *Sensory Integration and the Child*. Los Angeles, CA: Western Psychological Services; 1979.
2. Ayres AJ. *Sensory Integration and Learning Disorders*. Los Angeles, CA: Western Psychological Services; 1972.
3. Ayres AJ. *The Sensory Integration and Praxis Tests*. Los Angeles, CA: Western Psychological Services; 1989.
4. Su C, Parham D. Validity of sensory systems as distinct constructs. *Am J Occup Ther*. 2014;68:546-554.
5. Asher AV, Parham LD, Knox S. Interrater reliability of Sensory Integration and Praxis Tests (SIPT) score interpretation. *Am J Occup Ther*. 2008;62:308-319.
6. Dunn W, Brown C. Factor analysis on the Sensory Profile from a national sample of children without disabilities. *Am J Occup Ther*. 1997;51:490-495, discussion 496-499.
7. Mailloux Z, Mulligan S, Smith Roley S, et al. Verification and clarification of patterns of sensory integrative dysfunction. *Am J Occup Ther*. 2011;65:143-151.
8. Mulligan S. Patterns of sensory integration dysfunction: a confirmatory factor analysis. *Am J Occup Ther*. 1998;52:819-828.
9. Mulligan S. Cluster analysis of scores of children on the sensory integration and praxis tests. *Occup Ther J Res*. 2000;20(4):256-270.
10. Miller LJ, Lane SJ. Toward a consensus in terminology in sensory integration theory and practice: part 1: taxonomy of neurophysiological processes. *Sens Integr Spec Interest Sect Q*. 2000;23(1):1-4.
11. Miller LJ, Anzalone ME, Lane SJ, et al. Concept evolution in sensory integration: a proposed nosology for diagnosis. *Am J Occup Ther*. 2007;61:135-140.
12. American Academy of Pediatrics. Policy statement: sensory integration therapies for children with developmental and behavioral disorders. *Pediatrics*. 2012;129(6):1186-1189.
13. Parham LD, Cohn ES, Spitzer S, et al. Fidelity in sensory integration intervention research. *Am J Occup Ther*. 2007;61:216-227. doi:10.5014/ajot.61.2.216.
14. Parham L, Ecker C, Miller-Kuhanek H, et al. *Sensory Processing Measure Manual*. Los Angeles, CA: Western Psychological Services; 2007.
15. Parham LD, Roley SS, May-Benson TA, et al. Development of a fidelity measure for research on the effectiveness of the Ayres Sensory Integration intervention. *Am J Occup Ther*. 2011;65:133-142. doi:10.5014/ajot.2011.000745.
16. Watling R, Hauer S. Effectiveness of Ayres Sensory Integration and sensory-based interventions for people with autism spectrum disorder: a systematic review. *Am J Occup Ther*. 2015;69(5):1-12. doi:10.5014/ajot.2015.018051.
17. Mack W, Lindquist JE, Parham LD. A synthesis of occupational behavior and sensory integration concepts in theory and practice, part 1. Theoretical foundations. *Am J Occup Ther*. 1982;36:365-374.
18. Schaaf RC, Mailloux Z. *Clinician's Guide for Implementing Ayres Sensory Integration: Promoting Participation for Children With Autism*. Bethesda, MD: AOTA Press; 2015.
19. Florey LL. Studies of play: implications for growth, development, and for clinical practice. *Am J Occup Ther*. 1981;35:519-524.
20. American Occupational Therapy Association. Providing occupational therapy using sensory integration theory and methods in school-based practice. *Am J Occup Ther*. 2009;63:823-842. doi:10.5014/ajot.63.6.823.
21. Dunn W. Sensory Profile 2 User's Manual. Bloomington, IN: Pearson; 2014.

8 Cognitive Behavioral Models

Nature in her unfathomable designs has mixed us of clay and flame, of brain and mind, that the two things hang indubitably together and determine each other's being but how or why, no mortal may ever know.

—William James[1]
Principles of Psychology

Chapter Outline

Learning Objectives

1. Identify systems-level cognitive behavioral approaches.
2. State the key principles of the dynamic interactional model.
3. State the key principles of the cognitive orientation to daily occupational performance model.
4. Identify traditional performance-based approaches.

5. State the key principles of the neurofunctional approach.
6. State the key principles of the cognitive rehabilitation model.
7. State the key principles of the cognitive disability model.
8. Explain the influence of social cognitive theory on occupational therapy practice.
9. Outline ways that cognitive behavioral principles can be integrated into occupation-based models.

Key Terms

backward chaining
case formulation
cognition
cognitive disability model
cognitive orientation to daily occupational performance (CO-OP) model
cognitive rehabilitation model
dynamic interactional model
forward chaining
functional cognition
multicontext approach
neurofunctional approach (NFA)
perceived self-efficacy
self-awareness
social cognitive theory
whole-task method

Overview

Cognitive behavioral models incorporate certain basic concepts about thinking, learning, and behavior. Although occupational therapy (OT) researchers offer some variations, in general, **cognition** refers to the mental processes involved in perception, thinking, reasoning, learning, and memory. Cognitive behavioral occupational therapy approaches represent a broad perspective on factors that impact human performance, and as such, are not easily categorized into a single model of practice.

Principles from these approaches are applied across the life span and in every practice setting. The specific application of these principles differs on the basis of collaborative planning with patients and relevance-testing against expressed patient goals. Therapists may focus on a systems-level NOBA (not only but also) approach that addresses relevant impairments within a larger context of occupation.

Cognitive Behavioral Models and Occupational Therapy

Cognitive behavioral models in OT are based on the idea that cognitive processes have a broad and impactful relationship on behavior and participation in occupation. Cognition is defined as a process of taking in information for the purpose of synthesizing it and using it to affect behavior. Examples of cognitive processes include arousal, orientation, perception, attention, problem-solving, memory, and language use (Table 8-1).

An impairment in any cognitive process means that there is a strong likelihood that there will be a corresponding impairment with behavior. For example, a person with brain-injury-related memory problems could also have difficulty recalling the proper sequence for completing a morning self-care routine. Or the memory problems could affect the person's ability to function safely in a work environment. OT practitioners are interested in cognitive behavioral factors because of their influence on occupation.

To understand how occupational therapists incorporate cognitive behavioral factors into their work, we can think of these factors as *related knowledge* as described by Kielhofner.[2(p14)] He defined *related knowledge* as concepts and skills that are not unique to (OT) and not contained in specific OT practice models. Kielhofner recognized that cognitive behavioral knowledge from the field of psychology may sometimes be incorporated into OT practice.

Table 8-1
Cognitive Processes and Skills

PROCESS/SKILL	DEFINITION
Arousal	The state of being physiologically alert and awake
Attention	Ability to selectively focus and retain or release focus as needed
Executive function	A series of cognitive skills that refers to initiation, organization, sequencing, problem-solving, and decision-making
Language use	Using a system of symbols (verbal or written) for meaningful communication
Learning	The ability to acquire and retain new information that can lead to behavioral change
Memory	Drawing on or recalling past experience to use information in the present
Orientation	Awareness of self, others, and relationship to place and time
Perception	A process of recognizing and interpreting sensory stimuli
Praxis	The process of conceptualizing and planning motor action
Sensory registration	Detection of sensory information by the central nervous system
Visual scanning	Controlled use of the eyes to actively search the visual environment

Use of impairment-level cognitive behavioral approaches places the occupational therapist at risk of simply adopting the methodologies commonly used by psychologists, just as the use of impairment-level biomechanical approaches can look like physical therapy. However, there are times when those approaches are most appropriate for the context. Many occupational therapists using systems-level cognitive behavioral models are seeing greater research support for these methods.

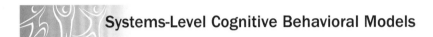

Systems-Level Cognitive Behavioral Models

Some occupational therapists have developed cognitive behavioral practice models that address a systems-level analysis of factors, in contrast to models that apply only to specific contexts. Systems-level approaches are frequently used in postacute contexts when more consideration is given to the individual's ability to engage with tasks in the environment, or more specifically, with his or her valued occupations. Systems-level approaches may be relevant in these situations because they tend to focus more on compensation and adaptation, as opposed to only remediation.

Table 8-2 provides a summary of the systems-level models discussed in this section.

Dynamic Interactional Model

The **dynamic interactional model**[3,4] is an example of a systems-level model. Reminiscent of the interactions described in Person–Environment–Occupation Performance models (see Figure 4-2), the dynamic interactional model describes how interactions between cognition, task demands, and the environment all influence occupational performance. Because of its alignment with existing occupation-based models, it is easily incorporated into these broad approaches to practice.

Toglia described some specific methodologies in her model, including a **multicontext approach** that uses an activity grading strategy for intervention planning. The individual is taught to use specific training strategies on the basis of assessment of fit between personal cognitive factors (including self-awareness), the environmental context, and task demands. This approach has been applied to children and adults with attention difficulties,[5] children with handwriting difficulties,[6] adults with traumatic brain injury,[7] and adults with schizophrenia.[8] This research underscores the broad way in which cognitive behavioral approaches are applied across the life span and in different practice settings.

Cognitive Orientation to Occupational Performance Model

The **cognitive orientation to daily occupational performance (CO-OP) model** is a systems-level model originally designed for children with developmental coordination disorder.[9] The model was developed in response to concern with component-level, bottom-up approaches. The CO-OP approach is performance-based, meaning that it focuses on competence in relevant occupational tasks (Figure 8-1). Once those goals are developed in

Table 8-2
Systems-Level Cognitive Behavioral Models

THEORY AND KEY READINGS	DEFINING FUNCTION	DEFINING DYSFUNCTION	ASSESSMENT	INTERVENTION
The dynamic interactional model had its first iterations in the 1980s and continues to evolve.[3,4]	The individual's ability to engage in task performance successfully Involves the use of information-processing skills and strategies to problem-solve and participate in occupations	The presence of any cognitive process or function that impairs performance Includes mismatch between personal factors, task elements, and environmental demand that interferes with the individual's ability to participate in preferred occupations.	• Static assessments: Standardized measures of specific cognitive functions • Dynamic assessments: Measures used to determine capacity for learning, including levels of awareness and strategies used • Toglia Category Assessment • Contextual Memory Test • Dynamic Object Search Test	• The OT practitioner grades activities and generalized learning in a multicontext approach in which the individual can learn to function under different demands. • Self-awareness training and promoting a fit between personal cognitive factors and environmental demand is emphasized. • Transfer of learning across environments.
The CO-OP model was initially developed in Canada for children with developmental coordination disorder, but is now being applied to a broad number of populations and has been adopted and researched internationally.[9,26]	The ability to use global cognitive strategies to facilitate transfer and generalization of learning for occupational performance	The presence of any cognitive process or function that impairs performance Includes mismatch between personal factors, task elements, and environmental demand that interferes with the individual's ability to participate in preferred occupations.	Assessments are used to help determine patient goals: • Canadian Occupational Performance Measure • Daily Activity Logs • Activity Card Sort • Pediatric Activity Card Sort Assessment is also directed toward observations meant to help prioritize areas for intervention: • Dynamic Performance Analysis	• Intervention is task-oriented and related to problem-solving by using self-talk, directed learning, and problem-solving for improving performance in patient-chosen tasks. • Goal-Plan-Do-Check is a global processing strategy that is used to guide performance during tasks. • Intervention should be fun, engaging, focused on independence, and directed toward generalization and skill transfer.

Abbreviations: CO-OP, cognitive orientation to daily occupational performance; OT, occupational therapy.

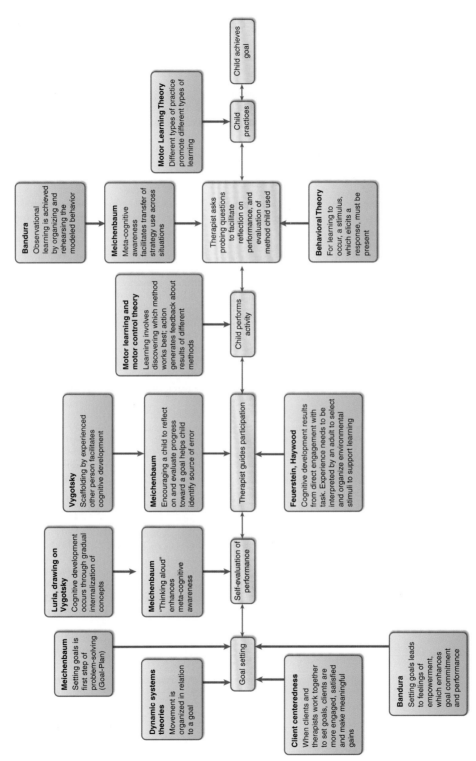

Figure 8-1 Theoretical basis and key components of the CO-OP model. CO-OP, cognitive orientation to daily occupational performance. (Reprinted with permission from Boyt Schell BA, Gillen G, Scaffa ME, et al. *Willard and Spackman's Occupational Therapy*. 12th ed. Philadelphia, PA: Lippincott Williams & Wilkins/Wolters Kluwer; 2013.)

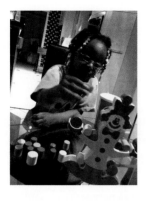

Figure 8-2   A young girl learns principles of balance through play with blocks of varying sizes and weights. (Reprinted with permission from Boyt Schell BA, Gillen G, Scaffa ME, et al. *Willard and Spackman's Occupational Therapy*. 12th edition. Philadelphia: Lippincott Williams & Wilkins/Wolters Kluwer; 2013.)

collaboration with the person receiving services, specific cognitive intervention strategies are employed to achieve goals.

Many CO-OP strategies are borrowed from cognitive behavioral theory, notably Meichenbaum's[10] Goal-Plan-Do-Check process:

1. The individual (and parent/guardian, if a minor) select a *goal* (or task) to be accomplished, and the therapist uses evaluation and assessments to determine if the goal is realistic and achievable.
2. The therapist performs a task analysis, and the individual and therapist collaborate to create a *plan* to reach the goal.
3. Using the planned strategies and methods, the individual works to accomplish the desired task or goal (Figure 8-2).
4. At a designated time, the plan is *checked* and evaluated to determine what worked, what did not, and what may need to be changed.

The individual is guided through a learning process that targets the strategies needed to gain desired skills. This approach qualifies as a systems-level method because of its attention to personal factors, task demands, and environmental influence (see Figure 8-1). The CO-OP model is easily incorporated into broad occupation-based models because of its close alignment with this Person–Environment–Occupation framework.

The CO-OP model has been expanded beyond its initial application and has been researched for effectiveness with many other populations, including children and adults with brain injury,[11,12] adults with age-related executive changes,[13] children with cerebral palsy,[14,15] and adults with stroke.[16,17]

Traditional Performance-Based Approaches

Traditional OT cognitive behavioral models are focused on performance-based strategies to improve targeted cognitive deficits. In these approaches, intervention is directed toward functional skill with arousal, orientation, perception, attention, problem-solving, memory, and language use. Therapists are incorporating more occupation-based elements into the descriptions of these models, making the distinction between *traditional* and *systems-level* models less notable over time.

Table 8-3 provides a summary of the performance-based approaches discussed in this section.

Table 8-3
Traditional Performance-Based Models

THEORY AND KEY READINGS	DEFINING FUNCTION	DEFINING DYSFUNCTION	ASSESSMENT	INTERVENTION
The NFA is mostly directed toward individuals with severe cognitive deficits. Although considered a *bottom-up* approach, it is still designed to ultimately attend to occupational performance.[18]	The ability to achieve the highest level of independent participation in occupational performance given the severity of cognitive deficits that may be present	A lack of task-specific training that causes increased disability, cost, and care burden related to people who have severe cognitive disabilities	Assessment begins with performance-based observations of whole-task functional activities without interference. Then assessment focuses on the subcomponents of cognitive performance. Samples include the following: • Test of Everyday Attention • Rivermead Behavioral Memory Test • Behavioral Assessment of Dysexecutive Syndrome	• Targeted skill retraining using the classic behavioral techniques of chaining, repetition, reinforcement, and graded support. • Skills are as generalized as possible across contexts and ultimately should reflect the preferred occupations of individuals who are receiving services.
The cognitive rehabilitation model is a traditional *bottom-up* model focused on remedial training strategies.[19]	Intact higher-order cognitive skill that can be used to functionally and adaptively participate in the environment	The inability to engage cognitive processes for adaptive functioning, including engaging in occupations	Assessment focuses on the subcomponents of cognitive performance. Samples include the following: • Loewenstein Occupational Therapy Cognitive Assessment • Dynamic Loewenstein Occupational Therapy Cognitive Assessment • Other standardized assessments of cognitive function Ultimately, performance in subcomponents is analyzed in the context of ability to participate in ADLs.	Intervention is designed to enhance residual abilities and to remediate areas of dysfunction. Includes targeted skill retraining through the following: • Paper-and-pencil tasks • Functional visual perceptual and visual motor training • Compensatory tasks • Computer-based training

(continued)

THEORY AND KEY READINGS	DEFINING FUNCTION	DEFINING DYSFUNCTION	ASSESSMENT	INTERVENTION
Cognitive disability model[21-23]	The ability to match and adapt cognitive skills for performing planned actions including normal activity demands and contexts	Impairment in cognitive processing that limits performance in sensorimotor processes, cognitive processes, and the ability to adaptively engage in tasks	Assessments are focused around skilled and structured observation of performance during designated craft or ADL tasks. Examples: • Allen Diagnostic Module • Allen Cognitive Level Screen • Routine Task Inventory • Functional observations	Intervention includes activities to improve normal cognition, to incorporate routine training, and to provide adaptations and compensations as needed.

Abbreviations: ADL, activities of daily living; NFA, neurofunctional approach.

Neurofunctional Approach

The **neurofunctional approach (NFA)**[18] is a bottom-up approach originally designed for individuals with severe cognitive impairments, particularly for those who might not benefit from a higher-level planning type of intervention, such as CO-OP. The NFA is designed to be occupation-based and integrated into a broader framework that moves beyond focus on simple or disconnected cognitive function.

There are eight stages to the rehabilitation process when using the NFA (Figure 8-3). The process begins with developing a strong and positive relationship with the patient

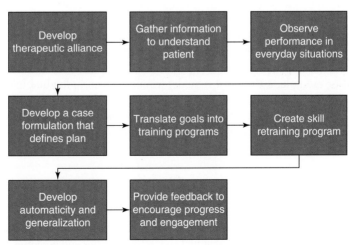

Figure 8-3   The eight stages of the neurofunctional approach. (Source: Clark-Wilson J, Giles GM, Baxter DM. Revisiting the neurofunctional approach: conceptualizing the core components for the rehabilitation of everyday living skills. *Brain Injury*. 2014;28(13/14):1646-1656. doi:10.3109/02699 052.2014.946449.)

and completing an assessment that includes broad data gathering and observation of daily living skills in the natural environment (as much as possible). Once that is completed, the therapist develops a comprehensive understanding of the individual's situation in what is called a **case formulation** (story), which is used to create a shared understanding of the situation. The case formulation is used to guide the treatment process.

The therapist works to develop collaborative goals that are continually confirmed with the patient, at his/her level of understanding. Skill retraining programs are developed in a planned, sequential manner that includes dynamic assessment of personal factors, task demands, and environmental context. Detailed task analysis and stepwise progression through sequential task steps is completed, preferably in a **whole-task method**, as opposed to **forward chaining** or **backward chaining** methods. Finally, those skills are generalized across contexts, and feedback is provided to encourage progress. This approach is generally most applicable with impairments that are severe enough to require a high level of task analysis, structure, and ongoing support.

Cognitive Rehabilitation Model

Similarly, the **cognitive rehabilitation model**[19] is a bottom-up approach that focuses on the development of discrete cognitive skills and then works toward generalization in more functional contexts. These types of approaches have been described in the OT literature for many years, including by theoreticians whose models began with this direct skill-training orientation but later developed into more complex systems-based approaches.[20]

The cognitive rehabilitation model is used with patients with a wide variety of cognitive impairments. Following an evaluation, the therapist works with the individual to strengthen intact cognitive skills, develop awareness of deficits, and use traditional intervention methods to train areas of weakness. It is common for intervention to initially take place in clinic-based settings. Traditional methods may not necessarily be occupation-based at the start of intervention but may take the form of paper-and-pencil tasks, visual perceptual and visual motor training, and computer-based training. These skills are reinforced and transferred to functional contexts later in treatment.

Therapists also use adaptation and compensatory techniques for daily activities. For example, a therapist may determine that an individual has visual scanning deficits and begin intervention using a computer-based game. Once the person develops some basic skill, those visual scanning abilities would then be transferred to more functional or occupation-based activities such as learning how to search a bathroom vanity for a toothbrush and toothpaste to complete morning routines related to the activities of daily living.

Cognitive Disability Model

The **cognitive disability model**[21-23] focuses on global cognitive processing as measured by *functional cognition* via structured tasks. **Functional cognition** refers to dynamic interaction between the individual's cognitive abilities and activities or performance contexts. The Allen Cognitive Level Screen is an assessment tool associated with this approach in which the occupational therapist observes completion of a craft activity. This assessment continues to be widely used by clinicians.

Level One

• Automatic Actions—Reflexive and basic function

Level Two

• Postural Actions—Basic gross motor skill and mobility

Level Three

• Manual Actions—Simple tool use

Level Four

• Goal-Directed Actions—Advanced tool use and basic learning

Level Five

• Exploratory Actions—Complex tool use, advanced learning, and socialization

Level Six

• Planned Actions—Typical functional cognition

Figure 8-4   Allen's cognitive levels. (Source: Allen CK, Blue T. Cognitive disabilities model: how to make clinical judgements. In: Katz N, ed. *Cognitive Rehabilitation: Models for Intervention in Occupational Therapy.* Bethesda, MD: American Occupational Therapy Association; 1998.)

This assessment methodology centered on concrete task performance may contribute to this model being categorized as *traditional*, but when used in combination with other assessments, including the Allen Diagnostic Module and the Routine Task Inventory, it is possible to create a comprehensive understanding of how cognitive disability is impacting occupational performance. On the basis of performance, a classification system (Figure 8-4) is used to identify patterns of performance, or cognitive levels. Once identified, the therapist works with the individual to improve functional cognition, and when necessary, also incorporates routines, adaptations, and compensations for occupational performance.

Social Cognitive Theory

Social cognitive theory is not specific to OT. It reflects the original work of Bandura,[24] who identified that there is a dynamic interaction between people, their behavior, and their environment. The fundamental premise of social cognitive theory is that people learn by observing others and that these observations can shape and change the way a person thinks. Bandura believed that although people learn as a function of their environment and their own personal factors, they are still capable of self-reflection and self-regulation. Concepts related to these ideas, such as **perceived self-efficacy**, are considered by many occupational therapists in their intervention plans. Perceived self-efficacy is what a person believes about his or her ability to perform.

Perceived self-efficacy was discussed by Gage and Polatajko[25] and later incorporated into some OT assessment tools. However, its relevance to performance (particularly as related to self-awareness and cognitive self-appraisal) makes social cognitive theory and perceived self-efficacy important concepts for therapists to understand and apply when considering cognitive factors that have a significant impact on practice.

Integrating Cognitive Behavioral Models Into Occupation-Based Approaches

The fact that traditional cognitive behavioral models persist is evidence that this type of intervention tends to be driven by the specific practice setting. For example, a patient in a critical care unit who had a brain injury may need to improve arousal level and basic ability to tolerate incoming sensory stimulation before addressing higher-level cognitive skills or more complex occupation. A preschooler with autism may require a gradation of food texture or tastes to learn how to tolerate changes in meals and the introduction of new foods. A young adult with intellectual disabilities in a transitional job training program may benefit from a backward chaining instructional approach to learn dressing skills. A middle-aged person in a rehabilitation facility following a stroke may need assistance with learning how to identify and use basic self-care items to overcome ideational apraxia.

These approaches underscore why traditional models still proliferate in practice. As occupational therapists became increasingly interested in adherence to core constructs of occupation, many of these models began incorporating reference to a more systems-level and occupation-based approach. However, the realities of practice settings and the acuity of patients' needs are pragmatic factors that influence intervention strategies.

The systems-level cognitive approaches take steps toward compliance with the NOBA methodology (Figure 8-5). Both the dynamic interactional model and the CO-OP

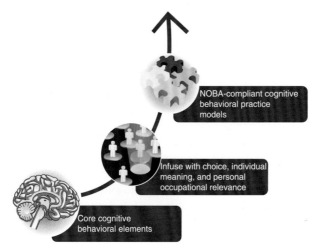

NOBA-compliant cognitive behavioral practice models

Infuse with choice, individual meaning, and personal occupational relevance

Core cognitive behavioral elements

Figure 8-5   Use of cognitive behavioral intervention strategies.

approach require patient-centeredness, consideration of complex interactions between abilities, tasks, and the environment, and a focus on meaningful occupation. Use of the traditional models requires more overt planning to ensure that the focus of intervention does not become restricted to the subcomponents of cognitive functioning at the expense of broader occupation.

CASE 8-1   *Michael*

Michael is a 19-year-old participating in a life skills and job training program during his extended high school experience. His diagnoses include monoarticular juvenile rheumatoid arthritis in his left hip and schizophreniform disorder (experiencing schizophrenia-like symptoms for less than 6 months). He is receiving consultative OT services as mandated by his Individualized Education Plan. The educational team has requested OT consultation to a paraprofessional job coach to facilitate the development of prevocational skills.

Motor Behavior

There are no overt motor difficulties, although Michael complains of occasional pain in his hip. He sometimes incorporates these physical sensations into complex delusional beliefs that he is made of robotic components that were implanted by the government. He ambulates stiffly, but functionally, and has a slow motoric response to functional demands.

Sensory Skills

Michael reports heightened sensitivity to light and sounds; as a result, he avoids as many social situations as possible. He uses isolation, rocking behaviors, covering his eyes, and headphones/music to block out the perception of unpleasant or intrusive stimulation.

Cognitive/Behavioral Skills

Michael is alert, oriented, and has functional communication skills. His affect and range of emotional response is flat. His attention was functional for short periods of time, but he reports having some difficulties with this. He cannot tolerate prolonged standardized assessment. There are no grossly evident deficits in sequencing, categorization, or other basic cognitive skills. He is capable of abstraction and concept formation, although several times during the assessment he interpreted statements literally. Michael has difficulty in developing operational strategies for addressing his perceived problems; in this sense he lacks in his learning and generalization capability, but primarily in social and emotive terms.

Summary of Cognitive/Behavioral Dysfunction and Impact on Occupation

Michael is able to express ideas and beliefs that have been inculcated by his family. He has a sense of morality that is so strong that he sometimes views situations in black-and-white terms. This causes him some difficulty, particularly when complex interpersonal relationships call for more nuanced interpretation, especially in high school social contexts. He expresses some *weariness* with what he perceives as chronic coping difficulties.

Michael has a wide range of interests, including golf and bowling. He reportedly enjoys solitary activities such as watching television and playing computer games. Socially, he has difficulty in the school context and rarely interacts with peers. He demonstrates poor coping skills and is dissatisfied with his ability to fit in. He remains unable to modify his behavior in response to environmental demands or in response to perceived parental aspirations. He often retreats into his own thoughts, which as previously identified, are sometimes reflective of delusional content. He is not interested in participating in the prevocational program.

Sample Goal From Intervention Plan

When given structure and supports, Michael will demonstrate the ability to identify personal goals related to prevocational participation and eventual transition to post-secondary-supported work environments.

Intervention Techniques/Equipment Used

The therapist might choose to follow a systems-level cognitive approach that can also incorporate the elements of social cognitive theory as well as occupation-based models. The first step is to guide Michael in a series of values and interest identification activities that reflect engagement of the volitional subsystem, as described in the model of human occupation (see Chapter 4). This process of values and interest identification will incorporate some important elements of social cognitive theory, particularly related to helping address Michael's deficits with perceived self-efficacy and fitting in with his peers. Using elements from a CO-OP model, the therapist can encourage participation in activities related thematically to current occupational interests and use graded exposure to new tasks for the purpose of exploration. Rank-ordering methodology can be used as an initial structure to promote decision-making. During this process, the therapist should attend to component deficits in attending, range of affect, and sensory tolerance. **Self-awareness** should be promoted through structured feedback sessions that point out challenges and incorporate positive behavioral supports and reinforcements for continued participation and learning. Ultimately, the therapist can guide these activities into relevant goals that are occupationally related and meaningful for Michael.

Sequence of intervention:

1. Collaboratively plan to identify meaningful goal areas.
2. Promote activation of interest through volitional subsystem.
3. Cycle through Goal-Plan-Do-Check methodology for addressing subcomponent barriers.

Analysis

Michael has an underlying capacity for participation in goal setting, but barriers related to his diagnosis and lack of skill in situational coping prevent his adaptive functioning. His symptoms should be monitored while engaging him in skill-building activities using a collaborative, goal-oriented, occupationally based method. With all of these aspects of his cognitive and behavioral challenges addressed, he is more likely to be able to continue development along an occupational choice process that can ultimately promote more competency and achievement behaviors.

Using the theoretical foundations, concepts, and assumptions inherent in cognitive behavioral models, do the following:

1. Review the case study and write a goal that you think may be relevant after 3 months of intervention. What skills do you think Michael can develop in that time frame? Include justification for your goal, a sequence of suggested intervention activities, and rationale for your choices.
2. Consider a situation in which Michael had an acute increase in symptoms and required hospitalization. In such a scenario, his cognitive ability could diminish significantly. If he was determined to be functioning at an Allen Cognitive Level Three (Manual Actions), was disoriented, and actively focused on delusional thoughts, how would his OT intervention be different while he was in the hospital? How would that impact your choice of intervention models?
3. List the advantages and disadvantages of using a *bottom-up* model of practice in which you focus first on the dysfunctional elements of cognitive performance and second on more broad occupation-based elements.

Summary

- Cognitive behavioral models are important in OT because cognitive processes have a broad and impactful relationship on behavior and participation in occupation.

- Cognitive behavioral OT approaches incorporate cognitive and behavioral factors into OT interventions to address specific physical, developmental, and psychological difficulties.

- Systems-level cognitive behavioral practice models include the dynamic interactional model and the cognitive orientation to daily occupational performance model.

- Traditional performance-based approaches include the NFA, the cognitive rehabilitation model, and the cognitive disability model.

- Social cognitive theory holds that people learn by observing others and that these observations can shape and change the way a person thinks.

- Cognitive behavioral models can be integrated into occupation-based approaches.

Reflect and Apply

1. Think of five different OT practice settings that you have personally experienced or read about. In what ways could cognitive behavioral approaches be incorporated into the care of people you saw at those locations? Were cognitive behavioral approaches actually used in each setting?
2. Working with a partner, complete a database search of a cognitive behavioral intervention that has good research support. Describe how that intervention method could be incorporated into an OT treatment session.
3. Working with a partner, complete a historical database search and write a brief analysis of how cognitive models have changed over time, including at what point there was evidence of greater consideration of occupation-based factors. Develop a hypothesis of why those changes occurred and compare your ideas with others in a group discussion.

Review Questions

1. Occupational therapists sometimes use information from other disciplines to inform theory development. The broad way in which occupational therapists incorporate cognitive behavioral approaches from psychology can be best described as the use of

   a. borrowed paradigms.
   b. related knowledge.
   c. general theories.
   d. occupational approaches.

2. Which cognitive behavioral model was initially designed as a bottom-up approach and eventually developed into a systems approach?

   a. Dynamic interactional model
   b. CO-OP model
   c. Cognitive disability model
   d. Cognitive rehabilitation model

3. Which practice model incorporates the cognitive behavioral strategies of Goal-Plan-Do-Check directly into its methodology?

    a. Dynamic interactional model
    b. CO-OP model
    c. Cognitive disability model
    d. Cognitive rehabilitation model

4. According to social cognitive theory, when an individual expresses doubt and concern with their ability to perform a task, they may have difficulties with

    a. internal locus of control.
    b. external locus of control.
    c. perceived self-efficacy.
    d. impaired self-monitoring.

5. Which model is most associated with assessment using specific task analysis of craft activities?

    a. Dynamic interactional model
    b. CO-OP model
    c. Cognitive disability model
    d. Cognitive rehabilitation model

6. All of the following are considered components of cognitive processes except

    a. arousal.
    b. attention.
    c. praxis.
    d. motor coordination.

7. The neurofunctional approach might be most appropriate for which patient?

    a. An elderly adult with traumatic brain injury and severe cognitive deficits
    b. A kindergarten student with mild autism
    c. An elderly adult with beginning memory loss
    d. A teenager with cerebral palsy and moderate intellectual disability

8. An important value of incorporating cognitive behavioral models into occupation-based models is

    a. greater patient collaboration for goal setting.
    b. greater likelihood of addressing impairment and functional concerns.
    c. greater likelihood of meeting relevant occupational needs.
    d. All of the above.

References

1. James W. *The Principles of Psychology*. New York: H. Holt and Company; 1890.
2. Kielhofner G. *Conceptual Foundations of Occupational Therapy Practice*. 4th ed. Philadelphia, PA: F. A. Davis; 2009.
3. Toglia JP, Golisz K, Goverover Y. *Cognition, Perception and Occupational Performance. Willard & Spackman's Occupational Therapy*. 12th ed. Philadelphia, PA: Lippincott Williams & Wilkins; 2013.
4. Toglia JP. The dynamic interactional model of cognition in cognitive rehabilitation. In: Katz N, ed. *Cognition, Occupation, and Participation Across the Life Span: Neuroscience, Neurorehabilitation, and Models of Intervention in Occupational Therapy*. 3rd ed. Bethesda, MD: AOTA Press; 2011:161-201.
5. Cermak SA, Maier A. Cognitive rehabilitation of children and adults with attention deficit hyperactivity disorder. In: Katz N, ed. *Cognition, Occupation, and Participation Across the Life Span: Neuroscience, Neurorehabilitation, and Models of Intervention in Occupational Therapy*. 3rd ed. Bethesda, MD: AOTA Press; 2011:249-276.
6. Josman N, Schein A, Sachs D. Use of the dynamic interactional model for handwriting intervention in children: explanatory case study. *Israel J Occup Ther*. 2011;20(1):E3-E27.
7. Zlotnik S, Sachs D, Rosenblum S, et al. Use of the dynamic interactional model in self-care and motor intervention after traumatic brain injury: explanatory case studies. *Am J Occup Ther*. 2009;63(5):549-558.
8. Josman N. The dynamic interactional model in schizophrenia. In: Katz N, ed. *Cognition, Occupation, and Participation Across the Life Span: Neuroscience, Neurorehabilitation, and Models of Intervention in Occupational Therapy*. 3rd ed. Bethesda, MD: AOTA Press; 2011:203-222.
9. Polatajko HJ, Mandich AD. *Enabling Occupation in Children: The Cognitive Orientation to Daily Occupational Performance (CO-OP) Approach*. Ottawa, ON: CAOT Publications ACE; 2004.
10. Meichenbaum D. *Cognitive-Behavior Modification*. New York, NY: Plenum Press; 1977.
11. Missiuna C, DeMatteo C, Hanna S, et al. Exploring the use of cognitive intervention for children with acquired brain injury. *Phys Occup Ther Pediatr*. 2010;30(3):205-219. doi:10.3109/01942631003761554.
12. Dawson DR, Gaya A, Hunt A, et al. Using the cognitive orientation to occupational performance (CO-OP) with adults with executive dysfunction following traumatic brain injury. *Can J Occup Ther*. 2009;76(2):115-127.
13. Dawson D, Richardson J, Troyer A, et al. An occupation-based strategy training approach to managing age-related executive changes: a pilot randomized controlled trial. *Clin Rehabil*. 2014;28(2):118-127. doi:10.1177/0269215513492541.
14. Cameron D, Craig T, Edwards B, et al. Cognitive orientation to daily occupational performance (CO-OP): a new approach for children with cerebral palsy. *Phys Occup Ther Pediatr*. 2017;37(2):183-198. doi:10.1080/01942638.2016.1185500.
15. Jackman M, Novak I, Lannin N, et al. Parents' experience of undertaking an intensive cognitive orientation to daily occupational performance (CO-OP) group for children with cerebral palsy. *Disabil Rehabil*. 2017;39(10):1018-1024. doi:10.1080/09638288.2016.1179350.
16. Ahn S, Yoo E, Jung M, et al. Comparison of cognitive orientation to daily occupational performance and conventional occupational therapy on occupational performance in individuals with stroke: a randomized controlled trial. *NeuroRehabilitation*. 2017;40(3):285-292. doi:10.3233/NRE-161416.
17. Wolf TJ, Polatajko H, Baum C, et al. Combined cognitive-strategy and task-specific training affects cognition and upper-extremity function in subacute stroke: an exploratory randomized controlled trial. *Am J Occup Ther*. 2016;70(2):1-10. doi:10.5014/ajot.2016.017293.
18. Clark-Wilson J, Giles GM, Baxter DM. Revisiting the neurofunctional approach: conceptualizing the core components for the rehabilitation of everyday living skills. *Brain Injury*. 2014;28(13/14):1646-1656. doi:10.3109/02699052.2014.946449.

19. Averbuch S, Katz N. Cognitive rehabilitation: a retraining model for clients with neurological disabilities. In: Katz N, ed. *Cognition, Occupation, and Participation Across the Life Span: Neuroscience, Neurorehabilitation, and Models of Intervention in Occupational Therapy*. 3rd ed. Bethesda, MD: AOTA Press; 2011:277-298.

20. Abreu BC, Toglia JP. Cognitive rehabilitation: a model for occupational therapy. *Am J Occup Ther*. 1987;41(7):439-448.

21. Allen CK, Earhart CA, Blue T. *Occupational Therapy Treatment Goals for the Physically and Cognitively Disabled*. Bethesda, MD: American Occupational Therapy Association; 1992.

22. Allen CK. *Occupational Therapy for Psychiatric Diseases: Measurement and Management of Cognitive Disabilities*. Boston, MA: Little, Brown and Company; 1985.

23. Levy LL, Burns T. The cognitive disabilities reconsidered model: rehabilitation of adults with dementia. In: Katz N, ed. *Cognition, Occupation, and Participation Across the Life Span: Neuroscience, Neurorehabilitation, and Models of Intervention in Occupational Therapy*. 3rd ed. Bethesda, MD: AOTA Press; 2011:407-442.

24. Bandura A. *Social Learning Theory*. Englewood Cliffs, NJ: Prentice Hall; 1977.

25. Gage M, Polatajko H. Enhancing occupational performance through an understanding of perceived self-efficacy. *Am J Occup Ther*. 1994;48(5):452-461.

26. Dawson DR, McEwen SE, Polatajko HJ, eds. *Cognitive Orientation to Daily Performance in Occupational Therapy*. Bethesda, MD: AOTA Press; 2017.

9 Motor Control and Motor Learning Models

The most important points in all of our developmental patterns are sequential order, activation for primary and secondary action in movement, and the resistance to stress. These apply to emotional, intellectual, and professional development as well as physical growth.

—MS Rood[1]

American Journal of Occupation Therapy

Chapter Outline

Learning Objectives

1. Identify traditional hierarchical control models.
2. State the key principles of the Rood approach.
3. State the key principles of neurodevelopmental treatment (NDT).
4. State the key principles of Brunnstrom's movement therapy.
5. State the key principles of proprioceptive neuromuscular facilitation.

6. Identify systems-level task-oriented models.
7. State the key principles of constraint-induced movement therapy.
8. State the key principles of task-oriented approaches.
9. Outline ways that motor learning principles and traditional and systems-level approaches can be integrated into occupation-based models.

Key Terms

attractor state
constraint-induced movement therapy (CIMT)
emergence
hierarchical control
hierarchy
learned nonuse
motor control
motor function
motor learning
muscle tone
reflex
reflex arc
release phenomenon
task-oriented approach

Overview

Occupational therapists must understand how movement occurs, how people learn to move, and how they recover that ability following damage to the central nervous system. As noted in Chapter 3, several physical and occupational therapists made important contributions to the developing body of knowledge regarding human movement in the 20th century.[2-4] The efforts of these therapists and many others reflected a reductionistic method of working to understand complex ideas by breaking them down into smaller parts. Over time, these initial approaches have been challenged by systems-level thinking that views human movement in much more complex terms. In this chapter, we will discuss both types of approaches to occupational therapy (OT) intervention.

Understanding Motor Function

Motor function is a general term used to refer to any movement or activity that occurs because of the activation of motor neurons. A **reflex** is a rapid action performed without conscious thought in response to a stimulus. The knee-jerk response shown in Figure 9-1 is an example of a simple **reflex arc**.

Many reductionistic therapy approaches were inspired by the work of Sir Charles Sherrington (1857-1952), an English neurophysiologist and physician who believed that reflexes were the basis for voluntary motor control. He explained that complex movement was controlled by a series of chain reflexes. This was initially a useful advancement in neuroscience but was only a beginning step toward a more modern understanding of the neurologic control of movement.[5]

John Hughlings Jackson (1835-1911) was an English neurologist who contributed important concepts that were later formulated into therapy approaches. He theorized that **motor control** occurs in a **hierarchy**, in which higher-level cortical centers exert command and control over lower-level midbrain and brainstem levels. Today, we describe this hierarchy as having three levels (Figure 9-2): the precommand level (highest), the

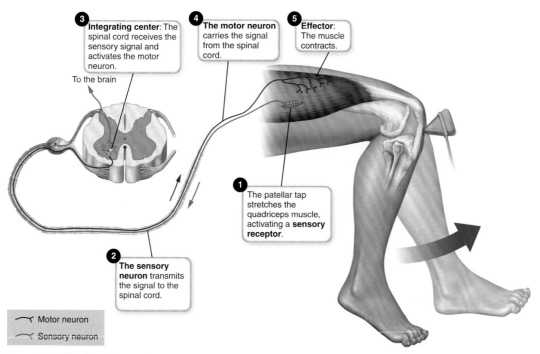

3 **Integrating center:** The spinal cord receives the sensory signal and activates the motor neuron.

To the brain

4 **The motor neuron** carries the signal from the spinal cord.

5 **Effector:** The muscle contracts.

1 The patellar tap stretches the quadriceps muscle, activating a **sensory receptor**.

2 **The sensory neuron** transmits the signal to the spinal cord.

⌒ Motor neuron
⌒ Sensory neuron

Figure 9-1   Simple reflex arc. (Reprinted with permission from McConnell TH, Hull KL. *Human Form, Human Function: Essentials of Anatomy & Physiology*. Baltimore, MD: Lippincott Williams & Wilkins; 2010.)

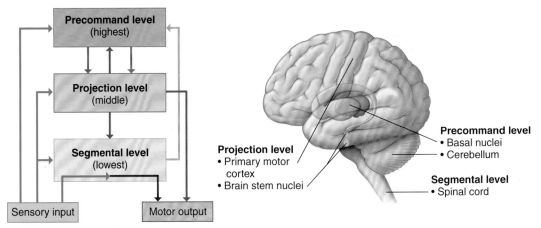

Figure 9-2   Hierarchy of motor control.

projection level (middle), and the segmental level (lowest). Jackson observed that reflexes from early phylogenesis (evolutionary development) were again present following central nervous system damage. His ideas about release of control and disinhibition from higher nervous centers formed the basis of early therapy approaches.[6]

Traditional Hierarchical Control Models

Applying the work of Sherrington, Jackson, and others, occupational and physical therapists developed treatment approaches that reflected the developing understanding of neuro-motor control. A model of normal motor functioning is depicted in Figure 9-3. Pioneering therapists developed treatment approaches that addressed dysfunction as it occurred within this model of normal movement. These approaches were a logical extension of reflex and **hierarchical control** models of movement. Margaret Rood, Berta Bobath, and Signe Brunnstrom made significant contributions on the basis of these ideas.

The basic premise underlying reductionistic approaches is that if the therapist focuses on the underlying cause of dysfunction, movement skill will improve. In simple terms, **muscle tone** can be normalized. Reflexive movement can be integrated. Weak muscles can be strengthened. Motor control can be developed. By resolving these kinds of problems in basic neuromotor function, there will theoretically be a corresponding improvement in functional skills.

The hierarchical therapy approach to promoting neurologic recovery was based on the observation of motor development in children and adults. A child normally progresses through sitting and standing and then walking as reflexive movements are gradually integrated into more mature movement patterns.[4] Following a neurologic injury, abnormal postural reflex activity results from the release of motor responses integrated at lower levels from the controlling influence of higher centers.[7]

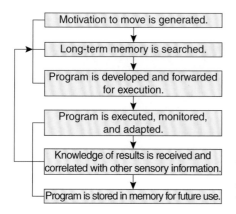

Figure 9-3   Reflex-hierarchical model of motor control. (Reprinted with permission from Radomski MV, Latham CAT. *Occupational Therapy for Physical Dysfunction*. Philadelphia, PA: Wolters Kluwer Health/Lippincott Williams & Wilkins; 2014. Originally adapted from Trombly CA. Motor control therapy. In: Radomski MV, Latham CAT, eds. *Occupational Therapy for Physical Dysfunction*. 7th ed. Baltimore, MD: Wolters Kluwer/Lippincott Williams & Wilkins; 1989.)

The underlying assumptions of these approaches include a belief that abnormal movement is the direct result of a neurologic injury that impacts motor control centers in the brain. For example, a blockage of the middle cerebral artery causes tissue death in the cerebral cortex. This, in turn, causes corresponding damage to neurologic control mechanisms. Because the cortex has inhibitory influence on lower brain centers, damage causes a **release phenomenon** and results in abnormal reflexive movement patterns that are controlled by lower brain centers.

Because reflexes and primitive movement patterns are developmentally modified and integrated into mature purposeful movement, restorative therapy was directed toward alternately facilitating and then inhibiting those abnormal movement patterns until normal motor control was reestablished.[2] For example, early in recovery following a brain injury, reflexes would be facilitated to promote muscle tone and basic movement responses. Later in therapy, the therapist would work to inhibit those abnormal patterns to promote refined movement.

Recovery was typically facilitated in a proximal to distal orientation. Flexion movements were promoted before extension movements, particularly in the upper extremities, and gross motor movements were facilitated before fine motor movements.[3] Proprioceptive and tactile stimulation was used to evoke changes in muscle tone and movement in selected muscle groups.[4] This pattern of working toward refinement and control of the motor system continued until satisfactory progress was achieved, or until the patient's progress plateaued. Table 9-1 summarizes key points related to the approaches described in the following sections.

The Rood Approach

The Rood approach[4,8,9] was an early sensorimotor model that was documented in Rood's early writings and then expanded on in OT textbooks. As such, there is not a lot of primary source material on this model. Four main components drive all assessment and intervention:

- *Assess available movement and then facilitate or inhibit movement responses using reflexes.* To accomplish this, therapists must be aware of the role that different types of sensory input have and how different sensory inputs can facilitate or inhibit

Table 9-1
Hierarchical Control Models

THEORY AND KEY READINGS	DEFINING FUNCTION	DEFINING DYSFUNCTION	ASSESSMENT	INTERVENTION
Rood approach[4] Neurodevelopmental treatment approach[7,10] Movement therapy[3] Proprioceptive neuromuscular facilitation[12,13]	Normalized participation in daily living activities that is achieved through typical neurophysiologic function and motor control	A primitive state of nervous system control that occurs because of neurologic injury and lack of typical command and control over lower brain centers	• Assessment of muscle tone, active range of motion, motor control, mobility, and other motor skills needed for occupational performance. • Most assessments are clinical/ observational and not standardized. • Specific observation guidelines are present for all of these approaches.	• Normalizing tone through inhibition and facilitation techniques • Inhibition or control of abnormal reflex activity • Facilitation of developmental motor control and postural reactions • Trial practice and training within the context of contextually relevant occupations and a more broad systems perspective has been added to the neurodevelopmental treatment approach as it has evolved over time.

movement. For example, light moving touch or tapping on a muscle belly would facilitate contraction of the agonistic muscle. Conversely, a prolonged stretch or the application of neutral warmth would inhibit contraction of the agonistic muscle.

- *Promote movement through developmental patterns.* Rood hypothesized that there were different levels of motor control: mobility, stability, mobility superimposed on stability, and skilled movements. The idea of incorporating developmental positions into intervention was to help the individual progress through these stages of normal movement development.
- *Promote purposeful movement.* Although Rood believed that movement could be facilitated developmentally, she identified that the end product of movement was application in a functional context. These ideas were expressed in broad terms of activities of daily living (ADL) participation, vocational capacity, and play (not in modern occupational terms).
- *Repetition.* Rood believed that purposeful skill was neurologically encoded following repetition and practice over time.

Although this model is not generally used in its entirety, the components of Rood's approach have influenced other traditional approaches that are still commonly used in clinics. Ideas about the facilitation and inhibition of movement are still applied in splinting and casting, as well as handling techniques described by Bobath. Additionally, Rood's ideas about developmental progression and levels of motor skill remain clinically relevant and applicable to modern practice.

Bobath's Neurodevelopmental Treatment

Neurodevelopmental treatment (NDT)[2,7] is a hands-on intervention approach to the examination and treatment of individuals who have movement and postural dysfunction caused by central nervous system dysfunction. These methods originated with the work of Berta Bobath, a physical therapist, and Dr Karel Bobath. They are based on the idea that a neurologic insult will lead to the release of lower-level centers from higher-level inhibitory control. This results in stereotypical postures and movement.

Early NDT focused on reducing muscle tone using reflex-inhibiting postures and sequential movement activities on the basis of normal development. Normal movement was facilitated and atypical movement was inhibited.

NDT has evolved significantly and has taken on many components of systems-level approaches.[10] In the past, NDT was oriented toward reflex and hierarchical models, but it now includes a view of the nervous system as a distributed heterarchy. Other changes include a focus on the importance of sensory input and feedback for motor control, and an emphasis on the importance of task goals and functional movement, as opposed to precision and quality based on muscle tone and postural responses. In using the NDT approach, the therapist is focusing on changing movement strategies to promote efficient movement that is functional and meaningful to the patient.

Current applications of the NDT model still incorporate an emphasis on precise therapeutic handling techniques, including facilitation and inhibition, to provide salient sensorimotor cues during functional movement (Figure 9-4).

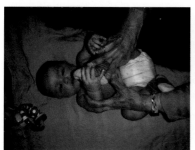 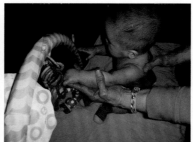 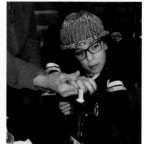

Figure 9-4   A therapist uses handling techniques and key points of control to help children of different ages develop motor skills. (Photos courtesy of Dee Berline, MBA, OTR/L, Therapy by Deesign, LLC.)

Brunnstrom's Movement Therapy

Signe Brunnstrom was a physical therapist who developed her Movement Therapy Approach[3] on the basis of the original work of Sherrington, Jackson, and others. As with other traditional approaches, Brunnstrom believed that normal motor development needed to be promoted following a central nervous system injury. She believed that recovery followed an ontogenetic process, meaning that regaining normal functional movement required progression through a sequence of stages.

The Brunnstrom approach was particularly helpful for clinical assessment and documentation because of the specificity in her identification of the stages of recovery (Table 9-2). She also promoted the use of proprioceptive and exteroceptive stimulation to promote and inhibit movements as needed. She believed that newly produced movements might first appear reflexively but required practice to be learned. She also believed that practice within the context of daily activities enhances the learning and recovery process.

Proprioceptive Neuromuscular Facilitation

Proprioceptive neuromuscular facilitation (PNF) is a treatment model developed by Herman Kabat, a physician, and physical therapists Margaret Knott and Dorothy Voss. It was originally designed to be applied to orthopedic conditions but later was also applied to neuromuscular dysfunction.

The PNF model[11-13] has an underlying philosophy that all people have potentials that are not yet fully developed and that goals should focus on abilities. The model's basic principles are that all normal movement should be spontaneous and that movements are both rhythmic and reversing in their character. These principles were applied by incorporating reversed movement patterns to establish or reestablish control of muscle groups. Postural reflex patterns were also used to initiate movement. For example, the asymmetric tonic neck posture would be used to promote wrist extension on the face side.

Table 9-2
Brunnstrom Stages of Recovery

STAGE	TREATMENT GOAL
1. Flaccidity	Promote movement
2. Associated reactions	Increase tension in muscles Attempting to gain synergies
3. Synergy	Voluntary control of synergies Initiating movement Increasing range of motion and strength
4. Declining spasticity	Reciprocal movements and mixed synergies
5. Complex movements	Willed movement with isolated control of muscle groups
6. Recovery	Recovery

PNF also follows a developmental sequence of movement recovery but adds complexity to functional movement by emphasizing the diagonal and rotary nature of mature movement patterns. These diagonal patterns are classified into flexion, extension, symmetrical, asymmetrical, and reciprocal components, which were incorporated into functional movement patterns, including ADLs.

Current Implementation

Reductionistic treatment models for neurologic rehabilitation are not being used as frequently as in the past.[14] This is partly due to the emergence of new theories and also for pragmatic reasons. Concerns about length of stay and increased requirements for focusing on functional skill acquisition for faster discharge impact models that therapists use. Additionally, as demands increase for evidence-based treatment decisions, therapists tend to abandon approaches that do not have strong research support. Despite these limitations, many therapists continue to incorporate elements of these models into their interventions.

Systems-Level Task-Oriented Models

The hierarchical view of motor control is inherently limited. Over time, researchers began studying broad ecological factors that influence human development.[15-17] Ecological and contextual theory development prompted a movement away from reductionistic models in many fields of study. As this influence reached motor control researchers, their work expanded beyond reflex and hierarchical control models for movement.[18-20] New models of motor control and **motor learning** shifted focus from the individual to the interaction between the individual and the environment. Experience-dependent neuroplasticity is the concept that the brain continually remodels itself in response to new information and contexts,[21] as shown in Table 9-3.

Expansive theories of motor behavior state that movement is the result of interactions between several subsystems that are constantly changing. **Emergence** refers to the occurrence of complex motor actions that result from the interaction of the person, the task requirements, and the environment.[22] Motor behaviors tend to self-organize on the basis of nonlinear dynamics; actions are constantly modified to meet environmental demand. Although varying situations require variability in motor behavior, patterns of movement tend to self-organize on the basis of expected conditions.

Significant neurologic deficit may cause motor behavior to self-organize into deep **attractor states** of reflexive, synergistic, and nonfunctional movements. Attractor states (preferred movement patterns) are not inherently functional or dysfunctional; rather, they represent stable efficiency states in which motor patterns tend to establish themselves on the basis of system constraints (Figure 9-5). For example, **learned nonuse** is when a person with a weaker extremity uses the stronger extremity to perform tasks instead of the weaker one because it is easier to do so. This phenomenon is an attractor state reinforced by a reduced use of the affected extremity during functional tasks, despite the contribution of

Table 9-3

Principles of Experience-Dependent Neuroplasticity

PRINCIPLE	DESCRIPTION
Use it or lose it	Failure to use functions leads to their decay.
Use it and improve it	Training and practice facilitates function.
Specificity matters	Specific training facilitates specific function.
Repetition matters	Practice is required for last change.
Intensity matters	Training intensity can also impact plasticity.
Time matters	There may be some criticality to timing for plasticity.
Salience matters	Training must be relevant to induce plasticity.
Age matters	Plasticity occurs more readily in younger brains.
Transference	Training in one area may enhance plasticity in another area.
Interference	Training in one area may interfere with plasticity in another area.

Source: Kleim JA, Jones TA. Principles of experience-dependent neural plasticity: implications for rehabilitation after brain damage. *J Speech Lang Hear Res.* 2008;51:S225-S239.

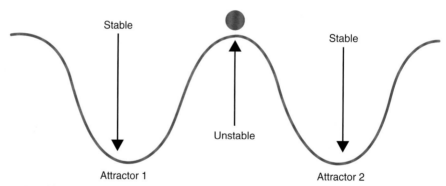

Figure 9-5 Motor behavior tends to self-organize into attractor states that are stable.

different sensory modalities and stimulation.[23,24] This cycle of nonuse is self-reinforcing and deepens the negative attractor state.

Table 9-4 summarizes key points related to the approaches described in the following sections.

Constraint-Induced Movement Therapy

These findings led to a new therapy approach of *forced use* or *constraint-induced* operant training to overcome the effect of nonuse.[25] **Constraint-induced movement therapy (CIMT)** approaches involve restraining an unimpaired extremity using a sling, mitt, or cast (Figure 9-6). The application of these devices, individually or in combination, restricts

Table 9-4
Systems-Level Task-Oriented Models

THEORY AND KEY READINGS	DEFINING FUNCTION	DEFINING DYSFUNCTION	ASSESSMENT	INTERVENTION
Task-oriented approach[35] Information processing model[20] Learned non-use model[25]	The expression of adaptive motor behavior that reflects adequate response to task and environmental demand	Inefficiency in movement that occurs when there are constraints on movements and inadequate affordance for compensation	• Assessment of muscle tone, active range of motion, motor control, mobility, and other motor skills needed for occupational performance • Task and environmental analysis • Most assessments are clinical/observational and not standardized.	• Constraint of the unaffected limb • Motor skills trial practice and training using designated operant protocols, practice schedules, and feedback mechanisms • Contextually relevant practice with skills that hold meaning and relevance to the individual

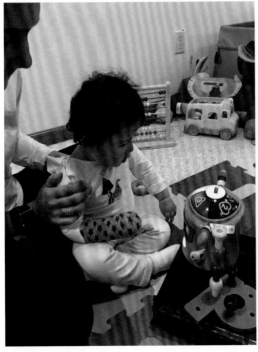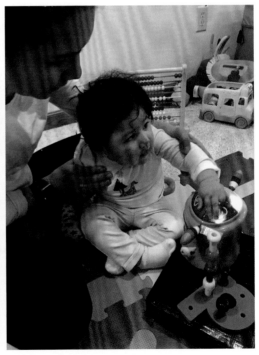

Figure 9-6   A therapist uses a modified constraint protocol with an infant who has left hemiplegia. (Courtesy of ABC Therapeutics.)

the use of the stronger extremity and forces the patient to use the impaired extremity. Improvements noted by using this method may occur because of mass practice with the involved extremity or through actual neurologic plasticity. There is not yet consensus on dosage, method of restraint, or eligibility criteria; there are still significant differences in the use of these protocols by researchers and clinicians. This method has been shown to be effective in progressively increasing function of the weaker extremity.[26-28]

In some CIMT protocols, prescribed practice opportunities are not always related to meaningful or functional tasks. Also, actual functional performance typically involves bilateral upper extremity (UE) skill. New research is beginning to address some of these concerns.[29,30]

Researchers are also beginning to learn more about the effects of interhemispheric inhibition, or the suppressing effect that one hemisphere can have on the other during neural reorganization following brain injury.[31] Transcranial direct current stimulation is a method of providing stimulation to the brain to mitigate the effects of interhemispheric inhibition. Some clinical trials demonstrate improvements in patients who received transcranial direct current stimulation along with CIMT protocols.[32] This has implications for clinical practice related to the use of stimulation itself, as well as protocols that promote unilateral versus bilateral training methods.

Task-Oriented Approaches

In contrast to hierarchical and CIMT approaches, some ideas from ecological theories have been applied specifically to therapy contexts; these are commonly referred to as task-oriented approaches.[33-35] This movement toward task-oriented approaches occurred in the context of the entire OT profession beginning to reconsider occupation-based models. In fact, PEO and task-oriented approaches have strong overlap and similarity (see Chapter 4).

The **task-oriented approach** includes training on specific functional motor tasks, developing practice schedules, and individualizing feedback to meet the needs of different learning styles. In collaboration with the patient, the therapist identifies control parameters that impact functional abilities. Those parameters might be patient-centric, environmental, or related to the task itself. With the help of a broad and comprehensive process of task or activity analysis, methods for relearning or adapting are employed for the patient to improve his or her functional abilities (Figure 9-7). A benefit of the task-oriented approach is that the patient is likely to be more engaged by a broad consideration of all these system elements. This leads to the likelihood of more practice, of higher contextual relevance of therapy tasks, and greater investment in problem-solving around areas of deficit.

Occupational therapists frequently include extra practice opportunities during their sessions with patients.[36] Random practice with high contextual interference is believed to be more effective than blocked practice.[37] Additionally, practicing movements as whole actions and in natural contexts (Figure 9-8) is believed to be more effective for training functional task performance.[38,39]

Unfortunately, the research controls required for the scientific study of motor learning compromise the real-life applicability of the interventions being studied. One criticism

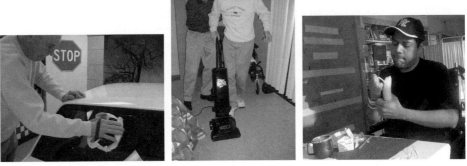

Figure 9-7   Examples of task-oriented activities. (Reprinted with permission from Radomski MV, Latham CAT. *Occupational Therapy for Physical Dysfunction*. Philadelphia, PA: Wolters Kluwer Health/ Lippincott Williams & Wilkins; 2014.)

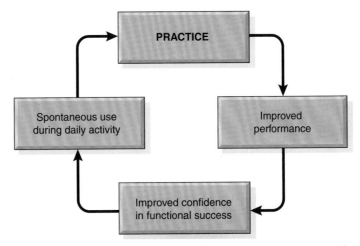

Figure 9-8   Repeated practice is used to promote long-term, continuous improvement in motor control. (Reprinted with permission from Radomski MV, Latham CAT. *Occupational Therapy for Physical Dysfunction*. Philadelphia, PA: Wolters Kluwer Health/Lippincott Williams & Wilkins; 2014.)

of some motor learning research is that it is often carried out using healthy individuals as subjects. Specifically, there are still many questions related to best methods for practice and feedback, particularly with populations of people who have neurologic damage.[40] Standardizing individualized and meaningful methodologies is challenging in the context of the actual variety of motor behavior that is observed in a clinical population. This complexity is amplified when applied to a population of patients who have unique neurologic problems that affect their occupational performance. OT researchers have made significant progress in studying motor interventions, but clinicians need to carefully consider research results when attempting to apply the available evidence to clinical decision-making.

Integrating Traditional and Systems-Level Models Into Occupation-Based Models

In clinical practice, occupational therapists use elements of both traditional and systems-level approaches. As noted for cognitive behavioral models (see Chapter 8), the demand for interventions is driven by the practice settings where occupational therapists work. For example, although the Bobath approach has been updated into a modern neurodevelopmental technique, it is not uncommon for a pediatric occupational therapist to employ specific inhibitory and facilitatory handling techniques when working with a young child with cerebral palsy. Using the approach this way does not ensure compliance with a NOBA (not only but also) methodology. Similarly, an occupational therapist employing a systems-level constraint protocol for an adult with hemiplegia does not guarantee that the methodologies employed include a patient-centered focus or meaningfulness for the individual.

Focusing only on the complex interaction between abilities, tasks, and the environment does not always lead to a patient- or client-centered approach to therapy. The use of both traditional and systems-level models requires patient-centered collaborative planning and consideration of personal meaning and contextual relevance to ensure that the focus of intervention is not restricted to the subcomponents of neuromotor functioning or motor learning at the expense of broader occupation.

CASE 9-1   *Ben*

Ben is a 67-year-old recently retired school bus driver. He had a right cerebrovascular accident (also called a stroke) that caused left hemiplegia (paralysis). He was initially hospitalized, and then, he spent 2 weeks in an acute rehabilitation facility. He has now been discharged home to the care of his family. He is being seen for occupational and physical therapy on an outpatient basis.

Motor Behavior

Ben can ambulate slowly with the use of a cane for support. He has an ankle-foot orthosis to control ankle positioning during gait. He requires supervision for stairs and uneven surfaces. Pain and lack of functional motor control limits his ability to reach and use his left arm functionally. He can close his left hand around objects, but edema and lack of sensory discrimination limit his function.

Cognitive/Behavioral Skills

Ben is alert, fully oriented, and there are no apparent cognitive deficits. He admits to feeling depressed about his situation, but he continues to have a strong interest in regaining his independence and organizes his daily activities to achieve that goal.

Summary of Neuromotor Dysfunction and Impact on Occupation

Deficits in motor control and coordination impact Ben with most of his daily activities. He requires moderate levels of assistance for personal care, including dressing and hygiene tasks. He has a strong desire to improve his independence with these tasks, but he is more concerned about needing assistance for meal preparation and self-feeding. Similarly, he has strong concerns about his inability to socialize. He previously enjoyed grilling and serving food and playing cards with his friends.

Sample goal from intervention plan: When given verbal prompts, Ben will stabilize a card holder with his left arm while reaching and placing cards with his right arm.

Intervention Techniques/Equipment Used

Engage Ben in preparatory mobilization activities, including passive and active assisted range of motion to reduce edema and pain in the left UE. Encourage UE weight-bearing for the facilitation of trunk control and proximal shoulder stability during functional ADL tasks. A trial of right UE constraint may be considered to encourage the increased use of the left UE. As intervention progresses, more time should be spent on task-specific training for occupations, such as using the left extremity to hold onto objects for purposes of stabilization. Opportunities for practice in natural contexts should be reinforced, such as during meals and card games with friends.

Sequence of intervention:
1. Collaboratively plan to identify meaningful goal areas.
2. Address underlying neuromotor deficits and learned nonuse.
3. Focus most intervention on trial practice and training for goal areas of high interest.

Analysis

The sequence of intervention for Ben is important to consider. Concerns about pain and lack of mobility need to be addressed first before he will be able to participate in preferred occupations. Addressing those components first will allow him some chance of functional participation in a constraint protocol. There is evidence to support preparatory and constraint protocols, but evidence also supports the primary use of task-oriented approaches using activities that are personally meaningful for the patient.

Using the theoretical foundations, concepts, and assumptions inherent in motor control and motor learning model(s), do the following:
1. Review the case study and write a goal that you think may be relevant after 3 months of intervention. Which skills do you think can be developed in that time frame? Include justification for your goal, a sequence of suggested intervention activities, and rationale for your choices.

2. If Ben does not achieve the baseline eligibility for participation in CIMT, what other methods might the occupational therapist consider to address concerns related to learned nonuse?
3. List the pros and cons of commonly used therapeutic exercise equipment such as an UE ergometer, weighted bars, and stacking cones as they relate to Ben's functional recovery.
4. Describe the expected outcome of the OT intervention process using motor control and motor learning principles.

Summary

- Motor function is a general term used to refer to any movement or activity that occurs because of the use of motor neurons.

- Treatment approaches evolved in the 20th century that reflected the developing understanding of neuromotor control based on hierarchical control models of movement. The Rood approach, NDT, Brunnstrom's movement therapy, and PNF are examples of traditional motor control models.

- The Rood approach was an early sensorimotor model that focused on regaining developmental control of movement and using specific techniques for the facilitation and inhibition of select muscle groups. Rood's ideas were incorporated in several other motor control approaches.

- Bobath's NDT was directed toward alternately facilitating and then inhibiting abnormal movement patterns until normal motor control was reestablished. It continues to be developed and now incorporates some systems-level approaches.

- Brunnstrom's movement therapy incorporated ideas of developmental control of function but is most notable for identifying stages of recovery that people commonly experience following neurologic injury.

- PNF is an approach that incorporates ideas of developmental control of function but is most notable for incorporating the use of archetypical diagonal movement patterns to facilitate recovery following neurologic injury.

- Later in the 20th century, motor control and motor learning models changed focus from the individual to the interaction between the individual and the environment; these models viewed movement as a result of interactions between several subsystems that are constantly changing. CIMT and task-oriented approaches are examples of systems-level models.

- CIMT approaches involve restraining an unimpaired extremity using a sling, mitt, or cast, which restricts the use of the stronger extremity and forces the individual to use the impaired extremity.

- Task-oriented approaches incorporate training on specific functional motor tasks, developing practice schedules, and individualizing feedback to meet the needs of different learning styles.

- The use of both traditional and systems-level models requires a patient-centered collaborative planning and a consideration of personal meaning and contextual relevance to ensure that the focus of intervention is not restricted to the subcomponents of neuromotor functioning or motor learning at the expense of a broader occupation.

Reflect and Apply

1. Reflect on OT practice that you have personally observed. Were the techniques that you saw reflective of more traditional or contemporary motor approaches? On the basis of your understanding of best practices, critique the methods employed and the progress that you observed.
2. Working with a partner, complete a database search of unilateral versus bilateral treatment approaches. Compare and contrast the approaches, considering a possible sequence for including both during intervention.
3. There is a lot of new research on the use of technology related to motor control and motor learning approaches, from the use of transcranial direct current electrical stimulation to the use of virtual reality and simulated environments for creating contextually relevant practice opportunities. How and why should these technologies be used by OT practitioners? Support your answer from a NOBA perspective.

Review Questions

1. Which of the following is *not* a common feature of reflexes?

   a. Reflexes are involuntary.
   b. Reflexes are unlearned.
   c. Reflexes are unpredictable.
   d. Reflexes are a protective response.

2. Which model best describes the *release* phenomenon associated with increased muscle tone and stereotypical posturing following severe traumatic brain injury?

   a. Contemporary motor learning
   b. Traditional hierarchical motor control
   c. NOBA
   d. None of the above

3. According to a 1996 study by Hanlon, which type of practice is most effective for retraining skills following neurologic injury?

    a. Random practice
    b. Blocked practice
    c. Random practice followed by blocked practice
    d. Blocked practice and random practice used interchangeably

4. Which of the following statements is true regarding attractor states?

    a. They are always dysfunctional responses.
    b. They are always functional responses.
    c. They tend to be energy inefficient.
    d. They tend to be energy efficient.

5. A child with cerebral palsy has spasticity in the right UE and trunk, poor head and neck control, and lack of mature postural reactions. These difficulties are limiting exploratory play behaviors and self-feeding. According to traditional treatment approaches, which problem would you address first?

    a. Right UE spasticity
    b. Inability to self-feed
    c. Limited exploratory play skill
    d. Delayed postural reactions

6. An occupational therapist instructs a parent to review the quality of a child's handwriting on a weekly basis. The use of this technique is consistent with which principle of motor learning?

    a. Blocked practice
    b. Random practice
    c. Providing feedback
    d. Positive reinforcement

7. According to the task-oriented approach, which factors are most important for a therapist to address when considering control parameters that are impacting motor behavior?

    a. Patient-centric factors
    b. Task-specific factors
    c. Environmental factors
    d. All of the above

8. An occupational therapist instructs a patient with a left hemiplegia to place a mitt on the right hand for several hours a day. This technique is referred to as

    a. constraint-induced movement therapy.
    b. the Bobath approach.
    c. the Brunnstrom approach.
    d. task-oriented therapy.

References

1. Rood MS. Every one counts. 1958 Eleanor Clarke Slagle Lecture. *Am J Occup Ther*. 1958;12:326-329.
2. Bobath B. The importance of the reduction of muscle tone and the control of mass reflex action in the treatment of spasticity. *Occup Ther Rehabil*. 1948;27(5):371-383.
3. Brunnstrom S. *Movement Therapy in Hemiplegia*. New York, NY: Harper and Row; 1970.
4. Rood MS. Neurophysiological mechanisms utilized in the treatment of neuromuscular dysfunction. *Am J Occup Ther*. 1956;10:220-225.
5. Molnár Z, Brown RE, Molnár Z. Insights into the life and work of Sir Charles Sherrington. *Nat Rev Neurosci*. 2010;11(6):429-436. doi:10.1038/nrn2835.
6. Franz EA, Gillett G. John Hughlings Jackson's evolutionary neurology: a unifying framework for cognitive neuroscience. *Brain*. 2011;134(Pt 10):3114-3120. doi:10.1093/brain/awr218.
7. Bobath B. *Abnormal Postural Reflex Activity Caused by Brain Lesions*. London, England: Heinemann; 1965.
8. Metcalfe A, Lawes N. A modern interpretation of the Rood Approach. *Phys Ther Rev*. 1998;3(4):195-212.
9. Rood MS. Neurophysiological reactions as a basis for physical therapy. *Phys Ther Rev*. 1954;34:444-449.
10. Bierman JC, Franjone MR, Hazzard CM, Howle JM, Stamer M. *Neuro-developmental Treatment: A Guide to NDT Clinical Practice*. New York, NY: Thieme Publishers; 2016.
11. Voss DE. Proprioceptive neuromuscular facilitation application of patterns and techniques in occupational therapy. *Am J Occup Ther*. 1959;13(4, Part 2):191-194.
12. Voss DE. Proprioceptive neuromuscular facilitation. *Am J Phys Med*. 1967;46(1):838-899.
13. Voss DE, Ionta MK, Myers BJ. *Proprioceptive Neuromuscular Facilitation*. 3rd ed. Philadelphia, PA: Harper & Row; 1985.
14. Umphred DA, Lazaro RT, Roller ML. Foundations for clinical practice. In: Umphred DA, Burton GU, Lazaro RT, Roller ML, eds. *Umphred's Neurological Rehabilitation*. 6th ed. St. Louis, MO: Elsevier; 2013:1-24.
15. Bronfenbrenner U. Toward an experimental ecology of human development. *Am Psychol*. 1977;32:513-530.
16. Gibson JJ. *The Ecological Approach to Visual Perception*. Boston, MA: Houghton Mifflin Harcourt; 1979.
17. Lawton MP. *Environment and Aging*. Monterey, CA: Brookes/Cole; 1980.
18. Bernstein N. *The Coordination and Regulation of Movement*. New York, NY: Permagon Press; 1967.
19. Latash M. *Synergy*. New York, NY: Oxford University Press; 2008.
20. Schmidt RA. *Motor Control and Learning*. Champaign, IL: Human Kinetics Publishers; 1982.
21. Kleim JA, Jones TA. Principles of experience-dependent neural plasticity: implications for rehabilitation after brain damage. *J Speech Lang Hear Res*. 2008;51:S225-S239.
22. Thelen E. Motor development. A new synthesis. *Am Psychol*. 1995;50(2):79-95.
23. Knapp HD, Taub E, Berman AJ. Movements in monkeys with deafferented forelimbs. *Exp Neurol*. 1963;7:7305-7315.
24. Taub E, Berman AJ. Avoidance conditioning in the absence of relevant proprioceptive and exteroceptive feedback. *J Comp Physiol Psychol*. 1963;56:1012-1016.
25. Taub E, Crago JE, Burgio LD, et al. An operant approach to rehabilitation medicine: overcoming learned nonuse by shaping. *J Exp Anal Behav*. 1994;61(2):281-293.
26. Amini N, Bagheri H, Abdolvahab M, et al. The effect of constraint-induced movement therapy (CIMT) on quality of life, function and range of motion of upper extremity of patients with stroke. *Mod Rehabil*. 2012;6(3):1-5.
27. Taub E, Uswatte G, King DK, Morris D, Crago JE, Chatterjee A. A placebo-controlled trial of constraint-induced movement therapy for upper extremity after stroke. *Stroke*. 2006;37(4):1045-1049.
28. Wolf SL, Winstein CJ, Miller JP, et al. Effect of constraint-induced movement therapy on upper extremity function 3 to 9 months after stroke: the EXCITE randomized clinical trial. *JAMA*. 2006;296(17):2095-2104.

29. Lee S, Kim Y, Lee B. Effect of virtual reality-based bilateral upper extremity training on upper extremity function after stroke: a randomized controlled clinical trial. *Occup Ther Int*. 2016;23(4):357-368. doi:10.1002/oti.1437.

30. van Delden AQ, Peper CE, Nienhuys KN, Zijp NI, Beek PJ, Kwakkel, G. Unilateral versus bilateral upper limb training after stroke: the upper limb training after stroke clinical trial. *Stroke*. 2013;44(9):2613-2616. doi:10.1161/STROKEAHA.113.001969.

31. Coslett B, Hamilton R, Hoyer EH, Celnik PA. Understanding and enhancing motor recovery after stroke using transcranial magnetic stimulation. *Restor Neurol Neurosci*. 2011;29(6):395-409.

32. Figlewski K, Blicher JU, Mortensen J, Severinsen KE, Nielsen JF, Andersen H. Transcranial direct current stimulation potentiates improvements in functional ability in patients with chronic stroke receiving constraint-induced movement therapy. *Stroke*. 2017;48(1):229-232. doi:10.1161/STROKEAHA.116.014988.

33. Almhdawi KA, Mathiowetz VG, White M, delMas RC. Efficacy of occupational therapy task-oriented approach in upper extremity post-stroke rehabilitation. *Occup Ther Int*. 2016;23(4):444-456. doi:10.1002/oti.1447.

34. Flinn N. Case report. A task-oriented approach to the treatment of a client with hemiplegia. *Am J Occup Ther*. 1995;49(6):560-569.

35. Mathiowetz V, Bass Haugen J. Motor behavior research: Implications for therapeutic approaches to central nervous system dysfunction. *Am J Occup Ther*. 1994;48:733-745.

36. Stewart C, McCluskey A, Ada L, Kuys S. Structure and feasibility of extra practice during stroke rehabilitation: a systematic scoping review. *Aust Occup Ther J*. 2017;64(3):204-217. doi:10.1111/1440-1630.12351.

37. Hanlon R. Motor learning following unilateral stroke. *Arch Phys Med Rehabil*. 1996;77(8):811-815.

38. Ma H, Trombly C, Robinson-Podolski C. The effect of context on skill acquisition and transfer. *Am J Occup Ther*. 1999;53(2):138-144.

39. Ma H, Trombly CA. Effects of task complexity on reaction time and movement kinematics in elderly people. *Am J Occup Ther*. 2004;58(2):150-158.

40. Fisher BE, Morton SM, Lang CE. From motor learning to physical therapy and back again: the state of the art and science of motor learning rehabilitation research. *J Neurol Phys Ther*. 2014;38(3):149-150. doi:10.1097/NPT.0000000000000043.

three

The Future of Occupational Therapy

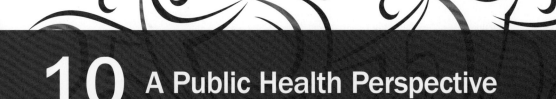

10 A Public Health Perspective

Beneficence is a duty. He who often practices this, and sees his beneficent purpose succeed, comes at last really to love him whom he has benefited.

—Immanuel Kant[1]
The Metaphysical Elements of Ethics

Chapter Outline

Defining Public Health and Population Health
Occupational Therapy and Public Health
Philosophical Concerns Regarding a Public Health Perspective in
    Occupational Therapy
Public Health and Social Justice Ethics
    Social Justice
A Public Health Lexicon for Occupational Therapy

Learning Objectives

1. Define *public health* and *population health*.
2. Describe how public/population health concepts relate to the practice of occupational therapy (OT).
3. Explain the concept of social justice and the ethical issues surrounding applying this principle to occupational therapy practice.
4. State the concerns associated with integrating public health/population health concepts into OT practice and ways these concerns could be addressed by the profession.

Key Terms

egalitarianism
population health
public health
social justice
Triple Aim

 ## Defining Public Health and Population Health

Public health has been broadly defined as "what we as a society do collectively to assure the conditions in which people can be healthy."[2] More recently, the Centers for Disease Control and Prevention (CDC) Foundation defined public health as "the science of protecting and improving the health of people and their communities. This work is achieved by promoting healthy lifestyles, researching disease and injury prevention, and detecting, preventing, and responding to infectious diseases."[3]

In the United States, public health management is part of the role of the CDC, a federal agency that is an operating unit of the U.S. Department of Health and Human Services. In addition, states and local municipalities have public health departments and agencies. The CDC's summary of the essential services of public health is shown in Figure 10-1.

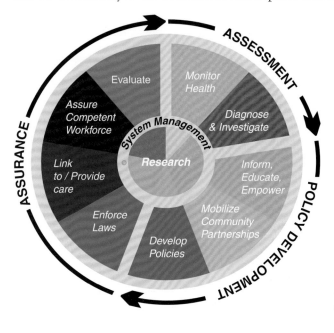

Figure 10-1   The 10 essential public health services. (Source: Centers for Disease Control and Prevention. The 10 essential public health services. https://www.cdc.gov/stltpublichealth/publichealthservices/essentialhealthservices.html. Accessed May 2, 2018.)

Population health is a term that is sometimes used interchangeably with public health. In 2003, Kindig and Stoddart defined the term as "the health outcomes of a group of individuals, including the distribution of such outcomes within the group . . . the field of population health includes health outcomes, patterns of health determinants, and policies and interventions that link these two."[4] Six years earlier, Kindig[5] had proposed the definition as "the aggregate health outcome of health-adjusted life expectancy (quantity and quality) of a group of individuals, in an economic framework that balances the relative marginal returns from the multiple determinants of health." This perspective was related to economics of care delivery and was included in methodologies to improve the U.S. health care system as defined by the **Triple Aim** of improving the experience of care, improving the health of populations, and reducing per capita costs of health care (Figure 10-2).[6] The Institute for Healthcare Improvement (IHI) is a nonprofit organization founded in 1991 on the basis of a commitment to redesigning health care toward these three primary goals.

Occupational Therapy and Public Health

Occupational therapists are proposing a role for the profession in public health/population heath. Leland et al[7] state, "Failure of the profession to clearly demarcate what constitutes high-quality occupational therapy and demonstrate its contribution to the broader patient outcomes that value-based care will measure may marginalize occupational therapy in the rapidly changing health care environment." These authors align the concept of value with the IHI's Triple Aim for populations.

Braveman[8] states that the occupational therapy (OT) profession should "identify specific competencies related to population health and public health and include them clearly in the Framework." Specifically, Braveman proposes an expanded role for practitioners that includes policy work for nonprofit organizations and/or federal health agencies.

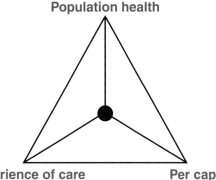

Figure 10-2   The Institute for Healthcare Improvement Triple Aim of health care. (Printed with permission from Institute for Healthcare Improvement.)

Philosophical Concerns Regarding a Public Health Perspective in Occupational Therapy

Adopting a public health or population health framework in OT requires a fundamental shift in philosophical orientation. Within a traditional framework of OT intervention, the focus and domain of concern center around the individual (patient or client). Due attention is given to levels above and below the individual because of their contextual relevance, but the primary scope of practice and domain of concern is at the level of the individual.

In shifting toward a population health approach, the primary scope of practice and domain of concern centers around the community. Public health/population health approaches are focused on broad community needs and frame concerns in broad population statistics.

There are several concerns with a shift of the OT domain of concern toward public health/population health. One of those areas of concern is based on a view of public health approaches as inherently paternalistic and not considerate of the needs of individual people in action who might instead be offered the opportunity to make autonomous and informed choices.[9]

Public Health and Social Justice Ethics

Public health is based on the ethical notion of **egalitarianism**, the idea that all people are equal and deserving of equal rights and opportunities. Most Western societies support this concept, but the means for achieving equality are hotly contested. Allowing for individual autonomy is often very challenging within a framework of egalitarian ethics. The traditional OT patient ethic is grounded in freedom and autonomy to self-determine quality of life. That principle is not always applicable in public health methodologies.

Social Justice

Occupational therapists' interest in population health is a fairly recent phenomenon. The 2010 American Occupational Therapy Association (AOTA) Code of Ethics stated, "**Social justice**, also called distributive justice, refers to the fair, equitable, and appropriate distribution of resources." The principle of social justice refers broadly to the distribution of all rights and responsibilities in society.[10] Interest in population health seems to be an application of the social justice construct, also deeply rooted in ethical egalitarianism. This concept has been incompletely defined as it applies to actual OT practice. Again, methodology of achieving equality is the primary point of contention.

The social justice principle was removed from the 2015 Code of Ethics. In part, its removal related to the difficulty in identifying what a violation of the principle would entail and how it could be enforced. The concept was not removed entirely; a reference to the social justice construct was included in the 2015 Preamble to the Code of Ethics, and the constructs of social justice and public/population health continue to appear in official AOTA documents.

Practical application of public health and social justice constructs remains unclear, primarily due to a lack of clarity regarding how "justice" is supposed to be operationalized as a treatment model. An entire issue of the *American Journal of Occupational Therapy* edited by Braveman and Bass-Haugen[11] was dedicated to social justice. Although there are some ideas proposed about using justice frameworks, these have not filtered into practice and there are pragmatic reimbursement and licensing issues that are barriers for such an orientation.

A Public Health Lexicon for Occupational Therapy

Clarification of salient issues must include definitions of assumptions, concepts, taxonomies, and subsequent research orientation; these are all critical for the evolution of concepts. The primary challenge in developing a public health lexicon for the OT profession is one of linguistics. Some linguists argue that a concept must be encodable for it to be stable. This is important so that the hearer can understand and form a mental concept of the message being communicated. However, other linguists argue that there are more concepts than there are encodable forms. In addition, it takes time for words to become established within a language.

Before trying to frame the nature of public health and justice for research and practice purposes, occupational therapists need to clarify concepts among stakeholders. This is important because as Kuhn[12] states, research is "a strenuous and devoted attempt to force nature into the conceptual boxes supplied by professional education." Unless the professional education is consistent and sound, the research that is conducted will be in danger of having serious flaws. This fact underscores the importance of having a well-developed lexicon; research will hold more value once definitions are broadly understood and accepted.

There is still some confusion as the profession begins to move toward a consensus opinion on the definition of public health and social justice concepts. Some theorists find that justice constructs have problems with logical coherence and systematization for practice.[13] These logical flaws need to be corrected before terminology is used as part of documents designed to guide practice and before therapists are asked to engage this model of practice. The broader implications of this problem are explored in Chapter 12 related to a fourth paradigm for the OT profession.

Summary

- Public health can be defined as the science of protecting and improving the health of people and their communities.

- Population health is sometimes used interchangeably with public health to refer to the health outcomes of a group of individuals.

- A public health/population health framework in OT requires a fundamental shift in philosophical orientation. Traditionally, the focus and domain of concern center around the individual (patient or client). Public health/population health approaches are focused on broad community needs and frame concerns in broad population statistics.

- The principle of social justice refers to the fair distribution of rights and responsibilities in society. Allowing for individual autonomy is often very challenging within a framework of egalitarian ethics.

- The primary challenge in developing a public health lexicon for the OT profession is achieving consensus on the definition of public health and social justice concepts and on how these apply to practice.

Reflect and Apply

Individual activities

1. The 2010 and 2015 versions of the AOTA Code of Ethics are available in the *American Journal of Occupational Therapy* online archives. Access these files and compare and contrast the two versions in regard to social justice and population health constructs. What are the differences and similarities? Do you agree or disagree with the changes?
2. Consider your personal values related to egalitarianism. How can the pursuit of equality be balanced against the rights of personal freedom in a democratic republic? How do you think the OT profession can operationalize public health concepts into a practice model?

Small-group activity

1. Working in small groups, research the definition of OT in the licensing laws of several different states. In a whole-class discussion, identify states that may or may not have difficulty with occupational therapists functioning from a public health/population health perspective.

Review Questions

1. Public health is best defined as
   a. what a society does collectively to assure conditions of health and safety.
   b. services to vulnerable populations that focus on eliminating disparities.

   c. clinical interventions provided primarily by nurses and governmental officials.
   d. a mandatory and integral function of every health care profession.

2. The IHI's Triple Aim of health care addresses all the following concerns *except*

   a. improving the experience of care.
   b. improving the health of populations.
   c. reducing the shortage of primary care providers.
   d. reducing per capita costs of health care.

3. Within a systems theory framework, the traditional domain of concern of the OT profession is primarily directed toward

   a. whole communities.
   b. families.
   c. individuals.
   d. whole cultures.

4. In the 2010 version of the AOTA Code of Ethics, social justice is defined as

   a. the fair, equitable, and appropriate distribution of resources.
   b. a core value of the OT profession.
   c. a governmental policy of wealth redistribution.
   d. an unenforceable and aspirational concept.

5. Identify one pragmatic barrier that makes implementation of justice approaches difficult in contemporary practice in the United States.

   a. Certification
   b. Licensing
   c. Accreditation
   d. All of the above

6. According to some theorists, applying justice concepts in OT is difficult because of

   a. a lack of systematization for practice.
   b. limited practitioner acceptance.
   c. limited regulatory acceptance.
   d. a lack of curriculum content.

7. What agency has primary responsibility for public health management related to the promotion of health and safety in the United States?

   a. Centers for Disease Control and Prevention
   b. Centers for Medicare and Medicaid Services
   c. Department of Housing and Urban Development
   d. Health and Medicine division of the National Academy of Sciences

8. In order for the OT profession to effectively adopt public health approaches, which of the following would have to occur?

   a. Inclusion of public health in the AOTA Practice Framework
   b. Inclusion of relevant exam content for certification
   c. Position papers published by reputable think tanks
   d. A shift in the OT domain of concern

References

1. Kant I. *The Metaphysical Elements of Ethics*. Urbana, IL: Project Gutenberg; 1780. www.gutenberg .org/ebooks/5684. Accessed May 19, 2018.
2. Institute of Medicine. *The Future of Public Health*. Washington, DC: National Academy Press; 1988.
3. Centers for Disease Control and Prevention Foundation. What is public health? 2018. https://www .cdcfoundation.org/what-public-health. Accessed May 2, 2018.
4. Kindig D, Stoddart G. What is population health? *Am J Public Health*. 2003;93(3):380-383.
5. Kindig D. *Purchasing Population Health: Paying for Results*. Ann Arbor, MI: University of Michigan Press; 1997.
6. Berwick DM, Nolan TW, Whittington J. The Triple Aim: care, health, and cost. *Health Affairs (Project Hope)*. 2008;27(3):759-769. doi:10.1377/hlthaff.27.3.759.
7. Leland NE, Crum K, Phipps S, Roberts P, Gage B. Advancing the value and quality of occupational therapy in health service delivery. *Am J Occup Ther*. 2015;69(1):1-7. doi:10.5014/ajot.2015.691001.
8. Braveman B. Population health and occupational therapy. *Am J Occup Ther*. 2015;70:1-6.
9. Buchanan DR. Autonomy, paternalism, and justice: ethical priorities in public health. *Am J Public Health*. 2008;98:15-20.
10. Beauchamp TL, Childress JF. *Principles of Biomedical Ethics*. 7th ed. New York, NY: Oxford University Press; 2013.
11. Braveman B, Bass-Haugen JD. Social justice and health disparities: an evolving discourse in occupational therapy research and intervention. *Am J Occup Ther*. 2009;63:7-12.
12. Kuhn TS. *The Structure of Scientific Revolutions*. 4th ed. Chicago, IL: The University of Chicago Press; 2012.
13. Hammell KR. Critical reflections on occupational justice: towards a rights-based approach to occupational opportunities. *Can J Occup Ther*. 2017;84(1):47-57. doi:10.1177/0008417416654501.

11 Occupational Science and Occupational Therapy

Attention to human suffering means attention to stories, for the ill and their healers have many stories to tell. The need to narrate the strange experience of illness is part of the very human need to be understood by others.

— Cheryl Mattingly[1]

Healing Dramas and Clinical Plots. The Narrative Structure of Experience

Chapter Outline

Basic and Applied Science
A Language of Occupation
Personal Context and Meaning
   Application to Practice
Systematizing Occupational Science Knowledge for Practice

Learning Objectives

1. State the goals and focus of the occupational science discipline.
2. Differentiate between basic science and applied science.
3. Describe various viewpoints regarding the relationship between occupational science and occupational therapy (OT).
4. Explain how key concepts of occupational science such as personal context have been applied in OT practice.
5. List the steps involved in a translational science research program and provide examples of this type of research.

Key Terms

applied science
basic science
ethnography
implementation science
occupational science
phenomenology
translational science

Overview

Occupational science is an interdisciplinary field engaged in the study of humans as occupational beings. It is focused on the form, function, and meaning of occupation. The field emerged as a means to help inform the occupational therapy (OT) profession, serving as a basic science for the applied therapy field.[2] The first occupational science department and degree program was founded by Elizabeth Yerxa at the University of Southern California in 1989. As a discipline, occupational science is still in its early stages of development. This chapter explores the evolving relationship between occupational science, OT development, and OT practice.

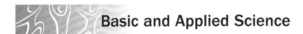 ## Basic and Applied Science

Basic science is defined as fundamental study with the goal of basic scientific discovery. Its purpose is to gain knowledge without concern for how this knowledge might be applied or used in the future. For example, occupational science research might include qualitative analysis of thematic elements related to the self-reported occupations of a subgroup of people.

Using a basic science orientation, an occupational scientist might interview an individual, analyze his or her writing, or use some other specific qualitative research method to better understand that person's lived experience and how the individual finds meaning in his or her occupation. The information thus gained would be used to understand occupation from a scientific perspective and would not be used to plan or implement therapy.

Applied science is the study and use of acquired knowledge to solve practical problems. OT is considered applied science because knowledge is used by therapists working with patients/clients to achieve mutually agreed-upon goals. For example, OT research might be conducted to determine whether a specific intervention was effective in helping individuals resume participation in occupations.

When the field of occupational science was established, some concerns were expressed about the birth of a basic science out of an applied field. Suggestions were offered for ways to meaningfully partition the basic science aims of occupational science from the applied science aims of OT.[3,4] The creators of occupational science responded that basic and applied science exist on a continuum and are not clearly distinguished from each other. They also argued that it was unlikely that occupational science research would lead to identity confusion among occupational therapists.[5]

Hinojosa[6] addressed the question of how the role of therapist and scientist differ. He stated, "The goal of all scientists is to add to the discipline's body of knowledge…. The goal of all occupational therapists is to assist clients to live more meaningful lives. When functioning as a therapist, the person's primary concern must be the client and addressing his or her needs. When functioning as a scientist, the person's primary concerns are investigating the phenomena of interest and maintaining the integrity of the selected method of scientific inquiry." Hinojosa concluded that although therapists could serve as scientists and educators, these roles cannot be performed simultaneously with the therapeutic role because of the incompatibility of the intent and methods.

A Language of Occupation

Occupational science is a developing discipline. Although many of its concepts are no longer new, they continue to change. Clarification of concepts, taxonomies, and research orientation are critical for the evolving discipline. There has been considerable debate among scholars, even in providing basic definitions for the concept of occupation. This is acceptable for a developing scholarly discourse but is less tenable for conducting applied research or explaining occupation to the public.

The evidence to date shows that there will likely be periods of confusion as the profession begins to move toward consensus on the meaning and definition of its central concepts. Yerxa[7] was concerned that "some might use such a lexicon to oversimplify and/or reduce rich, complex concepts . . . lead[ing] to premature closure of what should be a generative theory." Challenges with definitions persist two decades after she first expressed this concern.[8]

Classification systems must be understood as being conveniences that are subject to revision and debate. The developing taxonomies of occupational science can be considered a temporary and convenient filing system, not a set of fixed rules, until the field develops enough points of triangulation to create consensus. In practical terms, the developing lexicon used by occupational scientists might not always fit well within the constraints of OT practice models. Although occupational science research can inform OT practice, caution must be exercised in interpreting and acting on this information.

The following terms are mentioned throughout the occupational science literature. They represent ideas that are being explored by some occupational scientists, but they have not been consistently integrated into practice models for OT.

- *Occupational alienation* is a sense of isolation, powerlessness, frustration, loss of control, and estrangement from society or self as a result of engagement in occupation that does not satisfy inner needs.[9(p257)]

- *Occupational apartheid* refers to the segregation of groups of people through the restriction or denial of access to dignified and meaningful participation in occupations of daily life on the basis of race, color, disability, national origin, age, gender, sexual preference, religion, political beliefs, status in society, or other characteristics.[10(p67)]
- *Occupational deprivation* is the deprivation of occupational choice and diversity due to circumstances beyond the control of individuals or communities.[9(p257)]
- *Occupational justice* is the right of every individual to be able to meet basic needs and to have equal opportunity to reach toward his or her potential (specific to the individual's engagement in diverse and meaningful occupation).[11(p193)]
- *Occupational rights* include rights to meaningful occupational engagement, enrichment and growth through occupational engagement, choice, control, and autonomy around occupational engagement, and balanced occupational engagement with neither too much nor too little to do over a lifetime and in particular circumstances.[12(p67)]

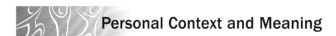# Personal Context and Meaning

Early outcomes of basic occupational science had direct correlation to practice. For example, many concepts from the new discipline emphasized personal contextual factors in OT. **Ethnography** is the scientific description of societies and cultures. Florence Clark's Slagle Lecture[13] introduced the concept of *individualized ethnography* to elicit personal contextual factors that can guide OT intervention. Clark noted that it may not be feasible for clinicians to conduct detailed ethnographies with their patients, but her case example provided a *thick description* through occupational storytelling and occupational story making.[14] *Occupational storytelling* is defined as a facet of clinical reasoning in which the therapist focuses on the patient's experience of a condition or disability to understand his or her situation in a personal and narrative context. *Occupational story making* is another facet of clinical reasoning in which the therapist and the patient create stories related to occupations that will be enacted in the future, organized around the new reality of illness, disability, or recovery.

Outside of the OT profession, cultural anthropologist Frank[15] and psychologists Polkinghorne[16] and Bruner[17] were advancing their own ideas about the use of narration to elicit life histories. These differing perspectives were brought together by Clark and ultimately influenced other researchers[1,14] who have made important contributions to occupational science.

Application to Practice

As an example of how this work relates to practice, Mattingly draws upon the expectation that current meaning is strongly dependent on a future sense of hope. She provides detailed analyses of therapeutic interactions between therapists and patients, providing examples of how therapists struggle against the notion that their patients with disabilities might experience time as a brute sequence of events. She shows that therapists work with patients to develop a shared vision for the future and of life after recovery from illness, injury, or disease.

Mattingly explains that the process of narrative within the context of therapeutic exchange may be construed as imitating the patient's life, or it may be that the patient's life is imitating the narrative being constructed between the therapist and the patient. She also proposes a third interpretation, suggesting that narrative imitates experience because of the therapeutic *sense-making* of the occupational therapist.

In the past 25 years, a plethora of articles and books have been published on the topic of personal contextual aspects that influence occupational performance. The idea of *personal meaningfulness*[2] is now frequently mentioned in the OT literature. Gray[18] proposed a methodology for considering occupations with the key premise that occupation cannot be interpreted separately from the person who is experiencing it, which is at the core of personal contextual meaning. She proposed a process of *bracketing*, in which a scientist would consider occupations first from a pure and unbiased perspective at each stage in a sequential process of philosophic inquiry (Figure 11-1). By engaging in this kind of analysis, her hope was that occupational therapists might be able to more fully understand the relationship between the individual and the person's occupations.

Hasselkus[19] devoted an entire book to the subject of personal meaning and occupation. Her text provides an in-depth study of how occupations must be considered within a personal context.

These contributions of occupational science applied directly to OT practice. All were notable for underscoring personal contextual concepts that were already partially expressed in Third Paradigm models, including the model of human occupation, but still not always applied in practice.

This basic research directly influenced some practice models that explicitly identified the relationship between the individual, the occupation being performed, and the environment. The Person-Environment-Occupation model[20] explicitly states that the behavior cannot be separated from its contextual influences. In addition, this model reintroduced the importance of history taking for establishing personal contextual relevance for goal setting.

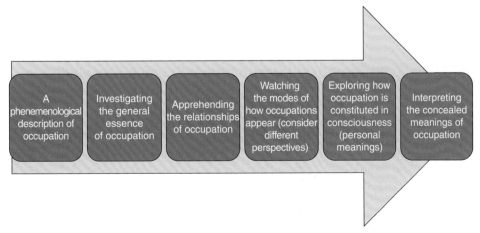

Figure 11-1   Gray's bracketing methodology for analyzing occupation.

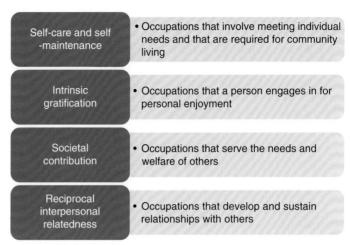

Figure 11-2   The four domains of the lifestyle performance model.

Similarly, the lifestyle performance model[21] took a congruent approach by embracing **phenomenology** (the study of a person's subjective experience) as the only possible method for understanding the personal contextual relationships between individuals and the occupations they engage in.

The lifestyle performance model is a methodology for understanding a person's occupations in full context of the person's environment and how he or she chooses to live. Quality of life is the central focus of the model and is defined in the context of harmonious life satisfaction in four domains: self-care and self-maintenance, intrinsic gratification, societal contribution, and interpersonal relatedness (Figure 11-2). This model is relevant in occupational science because of its emphasis on phenomenological reasoning related to the discovery of meaning in an individual's occupations and lifestyle. Additionally, Fidler[22] oriented her thinking about these concepts in ways that were intended to transcend application in a therapy context only.

Systematizing Occupational Science Knowledge for Practice

A model of systematizing occupational science knowledge for use in practice has been described[23] and is referred to as **translational science** (Figure 11-3). This translational approach involves seven steps that closely parallel a clinical decision-making process but also includes assessment of outcomes for an eventual purpose of theory development.

This translational approach has not been adopted by all occupational science researchers. Pierce[24] compares the American systematization that serves practice with the Australian model that "emphasizes occupation at the population level, the relation of occupation to justice, the need for policy change in regard to large-scale patterns of occupation, and

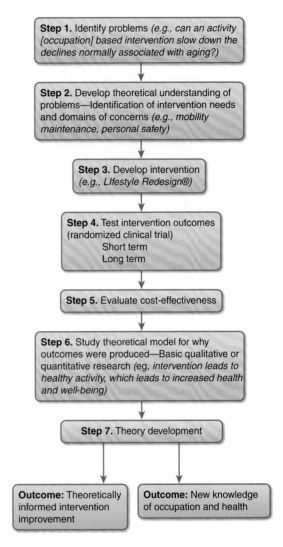

Figure 11-3   Blueprint for a translational science research program. Reprinted with permission from Boyt Schell BA Gillen G, Scaffa ME, Cohn ES. *Willard and Spackman's Occupational Therapy*. 12th ed. Philadelphia, PA: Lippincott Williams & Wilkins/Wolters Kluwer; 2013.

interdisciplinary research." These two different approaches to occupational science reflect some of the early concerns about whether the knowledge generated from this discipline would be basic or applied. Depending on the specific nature of the research, it has the potential to provide both types of knowledge.

Clark et al[25] describe the necessity of disseminating translational research for application to real-world clinical situations. They believe that there is a gap between the knowledge gained by researchers and the use of that information to inform practice. They propose using **implementation science** as a model, which focuses on promoting interventions that are clinically feasible, easily understood and implemented, and maintained by additional research and policy support.

Summary

- Occupational science is an interdisciplinary field engaged in the study of humans as occupational beings. It is focused on the form, function, and meaning of occupation.

- Basic science is research toward the goal of basic scientific discovery to gain knowledge without concern for how this knowledge might be used in the future.

- Applied science is the application of acquired knowledge to solve practical problems.

- Many concepts from the occupational science discipline emphasize personal contextual factors in OT.

- Clark introduced the concept of individualized ethnography to elicit personal contextual factors that can guide OT intervention.

- Gray's research methodology was based on the premise that occupation cannot be interpreted separately from the person experiencing it; she proposed a bracketing methodology in which occupations are considered at each stage of a sequential process.

- Basic occupational science research influenced some practice models that explicitly identified the relationship between the individual, the occupation being performed, and the environment, such as the P-E-O model.

- The lifestyle performance model incorporated phenomenology as the method for understanding the personal contextual relationships between individuals and the occupations they engage in.

- A seven-step model of systematizing occupational science knowledge for use in practice has been described and is referred to as translational science.

Reflect and Apply

Individual activities

In the following paragraphs, there are two journal entries written by the same man at different points in his life. The first entry, "My Hovel," was a reflection on his childhood. The second, "The Attic Bedroom," was a reflection from young adulthood when he was remodeling a home for his family. Read these entries and answer the questions that follow.

My hovel

I can't remember when I went to live in the cellar. In those days the seven of us shared three bedrooms. My brother and I had the bedroom off the kitchen, and the girls and my younger brother shared the back bedroom adjoining my parent's bedroom.

I had occasion to recall the furnace room where I lived recently in a conversation with my son. There was a coal box beside the boiler and although the boiler had been converted to oil before I moved in, still the coal box remained. And because the area of the furnace room where I lived had been a coal bin, I think for many years after I moved in, still the coal dust remained. No matter how I swept or washed, the coal permeated the walls and floor for years after the coal bin was removed. That may explain why I was able to commandeer this darkened end of the furnace room without much opposition from any other family member.

I just can't remember the early years in the furnace room. Like every occupation, I must have started off small and gradually expanded to fill the area of the old coal bin next to the boiler. There over the remaining coal box I placed an overhanging desktop and glass writing area. Later I built book shelves for the books I purchased from second hand stores in the city. I built a two by six plank workbench adjoining the coal desk along the back wall of the room and stored scrap wood for building under the workbench. I collected large dry cells from friendly telephone workers and made projects of simple electrical circuits. Years later it developed into a radio hobby, building power supplies and oscillators and studying code.

Through grammar school I would do homework, work at the workbench, and do carpentry work all through the evening hours. Every evening of the week was spent in my work area. The early years of photography developed in this area, and I remember constructing an enormous lateral enlarger from a large bellows camera. Although everyone lived upstairs, I lived in the cellar. And, I remember most how peaceful and quiet the furnace room was compared with the sometimes pandemonium upstairs.

The attic bedroom

You can't imagine how dirty and dark the attic on Orchard Street was when we bought the house. A winter clothes storage room had been built in the south wing of the attic below the high window, and the oversize beams supporting the slate roof were dirty and rough. A single light bulb hung in the middle illuminated the room and the upper half of the windows were colored glass, which permitted little light to enter the room on even the sunniest day.

Yet, the staircase was well constructed and the balloon construction lifted the perimeter walls 16 in off the floor in such a way that the sloped roof attic walls never seemed constraining, as attics often do. The center of the main section of the attic roof reached 14 feet off the floor, so that an 8-foot ceiling could be constructed through the large section of the room. The new Miami windows were installed from the inside of the room because the height of the house could not afford safe installation by ladder from the exterior. The electrical cable runs were over 250 feet of lighting and outlets, and I used 1,800 square feet of sheet rock over the insulation I installed. I think I taped the sheet rock for weeks.

(continued)

Before the floor was installed, my son wanted to move in, I think in 1970, he was only five. I bought the large IBM office desks from a moving company for 50 dollars each, including the swivel chairs. I piped the sink and waste to provide some relief for the busy bathroom on the second floor, which the six of us shared. Later I built the bookcases, which we promptly filled with a large library of collected books we loved. I remember how we loved to read the Reader's Digest Wonders of the World series. It became my favorite room, probably because I remember how dark, expansive, and dirty it was and later how airy, bright, and comfortable it became.

1. An occupational scientist (basic science) might be interested in analyzing these journal entries and identifying overarching themes to understand the development of occupations and meaning.
   a. Identify at least three different themes that are present in the two journal entries.
   b. How does this individual find personal meaning?
   c. How has this personal meaning been used to construct and influence his identity and parenting decisions?
2. An occupational therapist (applied science) might use these journal entries very differently to help develop an intervention plan.
   a. Describe how a NOBA perspective would be used to plan intervention.
   b. Write two goals that might be appropriate if this individual was unable to use one arm because of a stroke and was beginning to show signs of depression.
3. Consider the interests of the occupational science researchers described in this chapter. On the basis of your own observations and experiences, which occupational science ideas have the most application to practice? Explain how these concepts have been applied in practice and what outcomes you have observed.

Small group activities

1. Discuss whether it is important for all research related to occupations to serve the applied OT field.
2. Debate the concern about *resource drain* from the OT profession if some percentage of its academics pursue basic occupational science research. Consider the context of moving the profession toward a single point of entry at the doctoral level.

Review Questions

1. The original intent of occupational science was to
   a. provide basic science for the applied OT field.
   b. resolve conflicts between sociological and anthropological views of occupation.
   c. provide evidence-based practice recommendations for OT.
   d. encourage qualitative research in the OT profession.

2. An example of applied science in OT could be

   a. observation of rituals associated with parents dropping off children at school.
   b. research using narrative forms of diary writing to understand activity configuration.
   c. knowledge used by therapists to choose a specific evidence-based intervention.
   d. studying patterns of time use and activity choices among recent retirees.

3. Terms such as occupational apartheid, occupational justice, and occupational deprivation are

   a. being defined and explored for application to practice models.
   b. present in most major models of OT practice.
   c. universally reimbursed by commercial insurance plans.
   d. reflected in the core values of OT since its inception.

4. Other disciplines that have contributed idea to occupational science's focus on narrative inquiry include

   a. physical therapy and speech therapy.
   b. natural sciences and engineering.
   c. literature and fine arts.
   d. cultural anthropology and psychology.

5. Which process was proposed by Gray for scientists to study occupations in their purest forms?

   a. Personal interview
   b. Philosophical bracketing
   c. Quantitative research designs
   d. All of the above

6. The four domains of self-care/self-maintenance, intrinsic gratification, social contribution, and interpersonal relatedness are central to which model?

   a. Occupational behavior model
   b. Lifestyle performance model
   c. Model of human occupation
   d. Occupational adaptation model

7. An important contribution of phenomenology to occupational science has been

   a. emphasis on an individual's personal experience and meaning.
   b. added quantitative rigor to research methodologies.
   c. the introduction of general systems theory models to practice.
   d. All of the above.

8. Systematizing occupational science research for practice has been described as

    a. basic science.

    b. the development of grounded theory.

    c. translational science.

    d. participatory action research.

References

1. Mattingly C. *Healing Dramas and Clinical Plots. The Narrative Structure of Experience*. Cambridge, MA: Cambridge University Press; 1998.
2. Clark F, Parham D, Carlson M, et al. Occupational science: academic innovation in the service of occupational therapy's future. *Am J Occup Ther*. 1991;45(4):300-310.
3. Mosey AC. The issue is: the partition of occupational science and occupational therapy. *Am J Occup Ther*. 1992;46:851-853.
4. Mosey AC. The issue is: partition of occupational science and occupational therapy: sorting out some issues. *Am J Occup Ther*. 1993;47:751-754.
5. Clark F, Zemke R, Frank G, et al. Dangers inherent in the partition of occupational therapy and occupational science. *Am J Occup Ther*. 1993;47:184-186.
6. Hinojosa J. The issue is: therapist or scientist-how do these roles differ? *Am J Occup Ther*. 2003;57:225-226.
7. Yerxa E. Occupational terminology interactive dialogue. *J Occup Sci*. 1999;6:75-79.
8. Hammell KR. Critical reflections on occupational justice: towards a rights-based approach to occupational opportunities. *Can J Occup Ther*. 2017;84(1):47-57. doi:10.1177/0008417416654501.
9. Wilcock A. *An Occupational Perspective of Health*. Thorofare, NJ: Slack Inc; 1998.
10. Kronenberg F, Pollard N. Overcoming occupational apartheid: a preliminary exploration of the political nature of occupational therapy. In Kronenberg F, Algado SS, Pollard N, eds. *Occupational Therapy Without Border: Learning from the Spirit of Survivors*. Edinburgh, Scotland: Elsevier; 2005:58-86.
11. Wilcock A, Townsend E. Occupational justice. In Crepeau EB, Cohn ES, Schell BAB, eds. *Willard and Spackman's Occupational Therapy*. 11th ed. Philadelphia, PA: Lippincott Williams & Wilkins; 2009:192-199.
12. Whiteford G, Townsend E. Participatory Occupational Justice Framework (POJF 2010): enabling occupational participation and inclusion. In Kronenberg F, Pollard N, Sakellariou D, eds. *Occupational Therapy Without Borders Volume 2: Towards an Ecology of Occupation-Based Practices*. Edinburgh, Scotland: Elsevier; 2011:65-84.
13. Clark F. Occupation embedded in a real life: interweaving occupational science and occupational therapy: 1993 Eleanor Clark Slagle Lecture. *Am J Occup Ther*. 1993;47:1067-1078.
14. Mattingly C. The narrative nature of clinical reasoning. *Am J Occup Ther*. 1991;45:998-1005.
15. Frank G. Finding the common denominator: a phenomenological critique of life history method. *Ethos*. 1979;7(1):68-93.
16. Polkinghorne DE. *Narrative Knowing and the Human Sciences*. Albany, NY: SUNY Press; 1988.
17. Bruner J. *Acts of Meaning*. Cambridge, MA: Harvard University Press; 1990.
18. Gray JM. Application of the phenomenological method to the concept of occupation. *J Occup Sci*. 1997;4:5-17.
19. Hasselkus BR. *The Meaning of Everyday Occupation*. Thorofare, NJ: Slack Inc; 2002.
20. Law M, Cooper B, Strong S, Stewart D, Rigby P, Letts L. The Person-Environment-Occupation Model: a transactive approach to occupational performance. *Can J Occup Ther*. 1996;63:9-23.

21. Velde B, Fidler G. Lifestyle performance: a model for engaging the power of occupation. Thorofare, NJ: Slack Inc; 2002.

22. Fidler GS. The issue is: beyond the therapy model: building our future. *Am J Occup Ther.* 2000;54:99-101.

23. Clark F, Lawlor MC. The making and mattering of occupational science. In Crepau EB, Cohn ES, Schell BA, eds. *Willard & Spackman's Occupational Therapy.* 11th ed. Philadelphia, PA: Lippincott Williams & Wilkins; 2009.

24. Pierce D. *Occupational Science for Occupational Therapy.* Thorofare, NJ: Slack Inc; 2014.

25. Clark F, Park DJ, Burke JP. Dissemination: bringing translational research to completion. *Am J Occup Ther.* 2013;67(2):185-193..

12 The Globalization of Occupational Therapy

Globalization, or the increased interconnectedness and interdependence of peoples and countries, is generally understood to include two interrelated elements: the opening of international borders to increasingly fast flows of goods, services, finance, people and ideas; and the changes in institutions and policies at national and international levels that facilitate or promote such flows. Globalization has the potential for both positive and negative effects on development and health.

—World Health Organization[1]
Health Topics: Globalization

Chapter Outline

Learning Objectives

1. Explain how globalization has affected the occupational therapy (OT) profession.
2. Describe how international theory development has influenced American OT practice.

3. State the key principles of social and occupational justice approaches to practice.
4. Describe what is meant by a *fourth paradigm* in OT.

Key Terms

globalization
imperialism
occupational justice
ordinary meaning
sociopolitical determinants of health

Overview

Occupational therapy (OT) has experienced significant change over the course of its more-than-100-year history. Founding values that influence American clinical practice and resonate with U.S. practitioners were shaped by specific historical contexts.

The globalization of OT has generated a new wave of theory and model development that has provided the profession with a vision of practice that is unlike and sometimes at odds with the American philosophical foundation, which focused on autonomy and human agency. Global transference of OT models needs to be carefully considered because models are not automatically transferable to contexts where basic assumptions and concepts are not shared. This chapter explores paradigmatic changes associated with the globalization of OT and the emerging occupational justice and public health orientation.

Globalization and Change

Globalization refers to the spread of ideas, goods, services, and technologies around the world. In OT, it creates a challenge to the American understanding of how we define *community* in regard to practice and questions if we are all operating under the same set of professional values. Has globalization created a new OT paradigm?

Most OT practice in the United States remains aligned with models that reflect American sociopolitical contexts and educational/medical system values. Just as scholars from other countries note the challenges associated with integrating American theory into their local contexts, it is evident that there are similar challenges with integrating theory from other countries into an American context.

International Influences

Some OT scholars are proponents of the globalization of OT. Westcott and Whitcome[2] state that the holistic philosophy of OT "is not bound by national parameters." Concepts of social justice, equity, and meaning have been advanced as the global imperative of

OT educators.[3] Transnational advocacy networks have been proposed as the vehicle for developing a moral philosophy of the global OT community.[4]

New philosophies and frameworks are being advanced to move the profession in directions that will address 21st-century national and global problems believed to be associated with **sociopolitical determinants of health**,[5] which include disparities of power, ability, occupational participation, and many other factors. In advancing these new proposals, some scholars state that "ethical imperatives sometimes get bogged down in legal considerations of health care practice, as found in the United States."[6] At present, sociopolitical concerns are not designated domains of concern in OT licensing and practice in the United States.

Historical Context of U.S. Practice

Many occupational therapists in the United States continue to frame their practice around core values of the profession as established in this country. Change can be interpreted as problematic or evolutionary, depending on one's perspective. Paradigms change over time to reflect new research and new theories. However, when new theories are inconsistent with practice, this can represent a paradigm crisis.

What constitutes the **ordinary meaning** of OT for practitioners in the United States? Ordinary meaning is a legal concept that refers to the everyday definition and interpretation of a particular word, phrase, or idea. The statements of the American OT founders are best considered simply, directly, and in context with the profession's American heritage.

Recall from Chapter 3 that the OT profession experienced several paradigm crises in the 20th century. In the first paradigm (1917s-1930s), occupational therapists believed that occupation was important to human life itself. This philosophy was summarized best by Meyer,[7] who stated, "Our body is not merely so many pounds of flesh and bone figuring as a machine, with an abstract mind or soul attached to it" and that "Our role consists in giving opportunities rather than prescriptions. There must be opportunities to work, opportunities to do, to plan and create, and to use material." Much later, these values were echoed by Trombly[8] and Gray[9] in the frame of "occupation as ends and occupation as means." In essence, occupation is seen as both the goal of therapy and the method to achieve the goal. The values of the first paradigm were focused on health, skill development, and occupation.

In the second paradigm (1940s-1970s), occupational therapists were more likely to be concerned with occupation as an end and less often as a means. It was a time of interest in reductionism, and new core constructs emerged stating that performance is based on intact biomedical functions. The role of OT was to help people improve by addressing impairments. The values of the second paradigm were focused on internal systems, pathology, and symptom reduction.

Mary Reilly[10] proposed an occupational behavior model that promoted the concept that therapists should not only focus on biomedical science but also consider those factors within a larger focus on occupation. This model resolved the existing paradigm crisis. However, Reilly was concerned that American culture at the time might not be receptive to the idea of OT because American ideals related to productivity and mastery of the environment. She was not certain that therapists would be able to implement the concept of autonomy within a paternalistic medical system and wanted the profession to test her hypothesis about the action orientation and autonomy of humans. She explicitly stated that this hypothesis needed to be tested in an American context.

In 1980, Kielhofner and Burke[11] introduced the model of human occupation (MOHO), which incorporated many elements of the occupational behavior model. The following three decades saw a proliferation of theory development based around occupation-based models (see Chapters 4 and 5). The American concepts of volition, agency, habituation, and values surrounding work and human productivity are all woven into the fabric of MOHO theory.

Global Dissemination of MOHO

Although MOHO originated in the United States, Kielhofner's model subsequently spread around the world. Bowyer et al.[12] documented the extensive effort to disseminate these ideas, noting some cultural barriers, but identifying that "language is one of the most important barriers to dissemination." This may have been an understatement, particularly regarding the cultural specificity of the core concepts underlying occupational behavior, from which MOHO emerged.

During the period of rapid global dissemination, some authors began questioning the legitimacy of applying American theory in the contexts of other countries and cultures, labeling the practice a form of philosophical and theoretical **imperialism**. This criticism[13-19] states that the theoretical concepts inherent in a Westernized approach are inherently flawed, unscientific, and even dogmatic when applied in non-Western contexts. But Reilly had stated that her ideas reflected American professional values and that the theory was developed with the intention to test it in an American context.

It may be that OT is not a profession that can easily bridge different sociopolitical contexts, at least as originally conceived and as generally practiced in the United States.

Occupational and Social Justice

In the 1990s, the new discipline of occupational science emerged, accompanied by attempts at defining new *occupational* terms.[20] Thus, an entirely new lexicon was introduced into the OT field that included the concepts of social and occupational justice (see Chapters 10 and 11).

The **occupational justice** paradigm suggests intervention at higher levels of social and cultural complexity and endorses a model of distributive justice. Occupational justice and social justice are described as having in common concepts of equity[21] and the need for a just governance of society that promotes fairness, empowerment, and equitable access to resources.[22(p400)]

These new approaches emerged in part because of online and global communication methods that made collaboration and information-sharing easier among researchers and therapists in different parts of the world (Figure 12-1). Occupational science became a worldwide academic discipline.

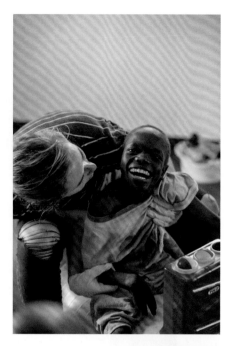

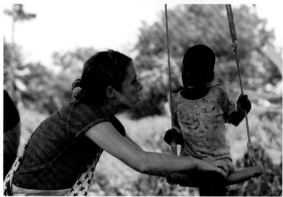

Figure 12-1   Clare Byrne is an American occupational therapist who graduated from Seton Hall University in 2012. In 2013, she had the opportunity to travel to Uganda, East Africa, where she spent a year volunteering her services to a population of children with severe disabilities. She returned to Uganda and in 2016 founded Imprint Hope, a nonprofit organization designed to raise awareness, break down barriers, and minimize the impact of stigma on children with disabilities. Many of the children she helps are marginalized and even mistreated. Her goal is to help each child and family realize a life of inherent worth, well-being, and happiness. The practical nature of occupational therapy takes on many meanings in a culture that is still developing and implementing policies related to health care and opportunities for children with disabilities. Occupational therapists who work in international settings must adapt their philosophy and methods to meet the needs of people as they are expressed in their unique contexts. Photos courtesy of Clare Byrne and Imprint Hope, www.ImprintHope.com.

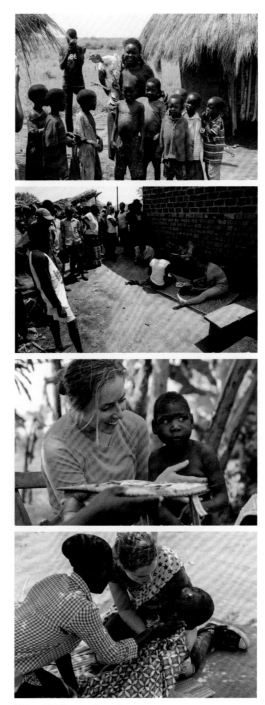

Figure 12-1   *continued*

Occupational science theory evolved differently in different locations. Pierce[23] explained the differences between American and Australian interpretations. American scholars largely sought to support the practice of OT and focused on outcomes research. Australian scholars sought to support their ideas on population health and the needs of a more socialized health care system. Pierce concluded that occupational science theory should evolve on the basis of research that meets the needs of practitioners, a perspective more aligned with an American viewpoint.

Some American OT leaders expressed strong interest in promoting a justice and population health framework that was being developed by non-American scholars. The Royal College of Occupational Therapists (U.K.) Annual Conference 2013 plenary by Iwama[17] discussed the concept that a public health model could make the OT profession more *relevant* for individuals and for society as a whole. These emerging values of social and occupational justice represent a very new paradigm for the U.S. OT profession.

Variance in the American Definition of Practice

Paradigmatic change began to be reflected in 21st-century American OT definitions. Over the course of a 12-year period, there was an ongoing redefinition in the AOTA Practice Framework. The original version stated that OT "focus[ed] on assisting people to engage in daily life activities that they find meaningful and purposeful. Occupational therapy's domain stems from the profession's interest in human beings' ability to engage in everyday life activities."[24]

The third edition (2014) states, "the clients of occupational therapy are typically classified as *persons* (including those involved in care of a client), *groups* (collectives of individuals, eg, families, workers, students, communities), and *populations* (collectives of groups of individuals living in a similar locale—eg, city, state, or country—or sharing the same or like characteristics or concerns). Services are provided directly to clients using a collaborative approach or indirectly on behalf of clients through advocacy or consultation processes."[25]

In just over a decade, definitions and methods of practice were described in dramatically different ways by the field's professional association. The definition had changed from a profession that meets the needs of individuals through occupation to a profession that also meets the needs of large groups of people through advocacy or consultation.

Wide variance in definitions of purpose inhibits the Framework's intent to clearly communicate the OT scope of practice to all stakeholders. It is important to consider if new definitions that emerge elsewhere in the world are compatible with American professional values and if such definitions can be implemented in actual practice in the United States.

Kielhofner[26,27(pvii)] expressed some concerns that there was a wide divide between theory and practice. He stated that he had ". . . increasing concern that the pendulum has swung too far in the other direction . . . that the field, in its eagerness to develop a science of occupation, may be leaving behind or forgetting the 'therapy' in occupational therapy."

Emerging Practice

Some occupational therapists in the United States continue to explore models of practice that reflect emerging paradigmatic values. Holmes and Scaffa[28] surveyed U.S. practitioners and found a lack of agreement about how to define *emerging practice*. Significant barriers were identified, including the lack of fieldwork educational opportunities and the lack of reimbursements. Some occupational therapists engage new paradigms in demonstration projects or proposals,[29,30] whereas others use paradigms to frame and describe theoretical constructs without actually engaging in the practice of OT.[31,32]

The number of American therapists working with new paradigmatic values remains low. Research indicates that fewer than 5% of all American clinicians work in *community* or *other* settings that are aligned with emerging practice paradigms and that these percentages have remained essentially unchanged since 2000.[33] These findings confirm that there remains a rather wide divide between theory and models promoted for practice and the reported practice patterns of therapists in the United States.

OT emerged out of a specific set of American social and cultural exigencies that are not present in these new definitions. The core values of autonomy and self-reliance resonate with most U.S. therapists. Despite being exposed to new values in the form of revised definitions of practice and mandated fieldwork based on justice and public health models, most American therapists still choose to practice using methods that align with what they see as their core professional values. Although all professions must evolve, it is likely that American therapists' fidelity to core values contributes to the low levels of adoption of methods labeled as *emerging practice*.

The Kawa Model

New models have been proposed that are intended to be more culturally relevant in different contexts around the world. One example is the Kawa model, which is described by Iwama[16] as an alternative methodology for conceptualizing a rehabilitation process. *Kawa* is the Japanese word for river, and the model uses this metaphor to explain a person's journey through life (Figure 12-2A). Water is equated with occupation, and the river's flow is congruent with well-being in life. Rocks represent challenges or problems, and driftwood represents personal factors that could impact or promote flow. The riverbed sides and bottom represent contextual influences that impact flow (Figure 12-2B and C).

The Kawa model is intended to be used for individuals, families, or larger collectives. It is not intended to provide concrete answers for specific clinical situations, but rather to facilitate a conversation in which the recipient of service can identify ways to achieve balance and harmony and allow the metaphorical river to flow toward its ultimate destination. This model has been introduced internationally and has generated broad interest, but it is not commonly used in the United States at this time, perhaps because of the rigidity of some of the systemic barriers that it seeks to overcome.

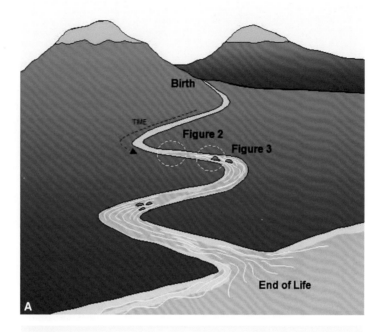

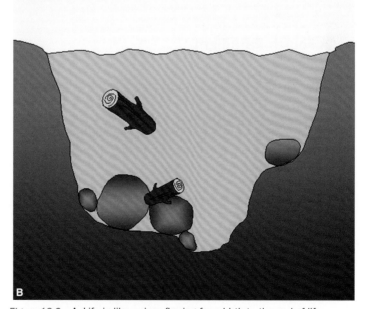

Figure 12-2   A, Life is like a river, flowing from birth to the end of life.
B, Basic concepts of the early Kawa model. C, The effect of river components
on flow. Adapted with permission from Iwama MK. *The Kawa Model: Culturally
Relevant Occupational Therapy*. Philadelphia, PA: Elsevier Limited; 2006.

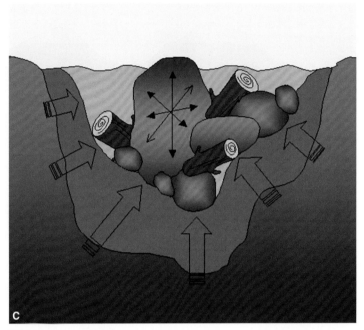

Figure 12-2   *continued*

A Fourth Paradigm

It is understandable that therapists in other countries who are unfamiliar with the American history associated with the profession's core values would approach OT practice differently, particularly in the context of their own social and cultural background. The creation of a fourth paradigm based on social justice and public health reflects a set of core values that differ from the original stated purpose of the American founders.

Just as American theory does not always philosophically align with the contexts of other nations and cultures when applied in these contexts, theory developed in other parts of the world does not always align with American contexts. Distributive and social justice interpretations may have more broad application in fully socialized health care systems or in different sociopolitical contexts. These models do not integrate well into the realities of American practice.

Social justice is not mentioned in the Values and Beliefs series,[34] and the notion of *justice* was not a driving philosophical point in regard to the profession's U.S. origins. This does not absolutely preclude practice using justice-oriented models in the United States, but it explains why most practice in the United States remains in alignment with the original American core values.

Reed[35(p78)] stated, "The models that seem to offer the best frame of reference for occupational therapy all come from the organismic meta model. Those from the mechanistic meta model such as the biomedical and public health models, do not provide a workable frame of reference for occupational therapy because the philosophy is counter to the beliefs and values on which occupational therapy was founded." Public health, like social justice, is based on the notion of egalitarianism. Application and respect for autonomy is often very challenging within a public health context. How can new justice models square with American theory that is oriented more specifically around the nature of human autonomy?

Admittedly, there is not absolute agreement in regard to American core professional values, and some therapists may prefer emerging models, but there is a reason why emerging practice paradigms based on social justice and population health do not resonate with the majority of occupational therapists in the United States.

Summary

- Globalization refers to the spread of ideas, goods, services, and technologies around the world.

- Most OT practice in the United States is aligned with models that reflect American sociopolitical contexts and educational/medical system values.

- New philosophies and frameworks have emerged and these are designed to address 21st-century national and global problems associated with the sociopolitical determinants of health.

- The occupational justice paradigm suggests intervention at higher levels of social and cultural complexity.

- Occupational justice and social justice share common concepts of equity and the promotion of fairness, empowerment, and equal access to resources.

- American theory does not always philosophically align with the contexts of other nations and cultures when applied in these contexts, theory developed in other parts of the world does not always align with American contexts.

- Distributive and social justice interpretations may have more broad application in fully socialized health care systems or in different sociopolitical contexts than those in the United States.

Reflect and Apply

Individual activities

1. Read Reed's Core Values and Beliefs series.[34] Consider how the values and beliefs documented at the time of the profession's founding align with emerging ideas about occupational and social justice.
2. Using the ideas expressed in the Kawa model, draw a picture of your own *river* and identify rocks, driftwood, and riverbed sides and bottom that are impacting your occupational *flow*.

Small-group activity

1. Research the basis of practice of OT in several other countries and interact with practitioners from those countries in professional forums or on social media. In a small-group discussion, consider the question: To what extent, if any, is OT a unified profession as practiced around the world?

Review Questions

1. Globalization in OT was primarily achieved through

   a. increase in international communication online and via other methods.
   b. mandated participation in the World Federation of Occupational Therapy.
   c. the creation of worldwide certification standards.
   d. the creation of more international OT journals.

2. Issues related to power and economic disparities and the ability to engage in meaningful occupations are sometimes framed by occupational therapists as

   a. occupational discrimination.
   b. environmental determinants of health.
   c. sociopolitical determinants of health.
   d. racial discrimination.

3. First paradigm values in an American context are best characterized as

   a. occupation as ends.
   b. occupation as means.
   c. occupation as both ends and means.
   d. occupation as neither ends nor means.

4. Mary Reilly explicitly stated that she intended for OT theoretical constructs to be applied and evaluated in

   a. only Western contexts.
   b. an American context.
   c. an international context.
   d. both American and international contexts.

5. Occupational and social justice have common elements, including the promotion of

   a. the values of independence and self-determination.
   b. individual responsibility for resource allocation.

    c. political methodologies for autocratic governance.

    d. fairness, empowerment, and equitable access to resources.

6. The use of models created in Western contexts that are not culturally relevant in other countries is called

    a. theoretical imperialism.

    b. occupational injustice.

    c. social injustice.

    d. occupational apartheid.

7. Which concept was *not* discussed in Reed's Values and Beliefs series?

    a. Moral treatment

    b. Social justice

    c. Pragmatism

    d. Therapeutic occupation

8. In the Kawa model, which metaphorical element represents harmony and balance?

    a. The rocks that create natural barriers in a person's life

    b. The driftwood that can knock down barriers and promote flow

    c. The mountaintop where the water originates

    d. The relationship of the water's flow to the riverbed and its contents

References

1. World Health Organization. Health topics: globalization. 2018. http://www.who.int/topics/globalization/en/. Accessed May 15, 2018.
2. Westcott L, Whitcombe SW. Globalisation and occupational therapy: poles apart? *Br J Occup Ther.* 2003;66(7):328-330.
3. Thibeault R. Globalisation, universities and the future of occupational therapy: dispatches for the majority world. *Aust Occup Ther J.* 2006;53(3):159-165.
4. Frank G. The 2010 Ruth Zemke Lecture in occupational science occupational therapy/occupational science/occupational justice: moral commitments and global assemblages. *J Occup Sci.* 2012;19(1):25-35.
5. Pollard N, Sakellariou D, Kronenberg F. *A Political Practice of Occupational Therapy.* Edinburgh, Scotland: Churchill-Livingstone; 2009.
6. Taff SD, Bakhshi P, Babulal GM. The accountability-well-being-ethics framework: a new philosophical foundation for occupational therapy. *Can J Occup Ther. Revue Canadienne D'ergothérapie.* 2014;81(5):320-329.
7. Meyer A. The philosophy of occupational therapy. *Arch Occup Ther.* 1922;1:1-10.
8. Trombly CA. The 1995 Eleanor Clarke Slagle Lecture: occupation: purposefulness and meaningfulness as therapeutic mechanisms. *Am J Occup Ther.* 1995;49:960-972.
9. Gray JM. Putting occupation into practice: occupation as ends, occupation as means. *Am J Occup Ther.* 1998;52:354-365.
10. Reilly M. Occupational therapy can be one of the great ideas of 20th century medicine. *Am J Occup Ther.* 1962;16:2-9.

11. Kielhofner G, Burke JP. A model of human occupation, part 1. Conceptual framework and content. *Am J Occup Ther*. 1980;34(9):572-581.

12. Bowyer P, Belanger R, Briand C, et al. International efforts to disseminate and develop the model of human occupation. *Occup Ther Health Care*. 2008;22:1-24.

13. Mocellin G. An overview of occupational therapy in the context of the American influence on the profession, Parts 1 and 2. *Br J Occup Ther*. 1992;55(1-2):7-12:55-60.

14. Mocellin G. Occupational therapy: a critical overview, Part 1. *Br J Occup Ther*. 1995;58(12):502-506.

15. Mocellin G. Occupational therapy: a critical overview, Part 2. *Br J Occup Ther*. 1996;59(1):11-16.

16. Iwama MK. *The Kawa Model: Culturally Relevant Occupational Therapy*. Edinburgh, Scotland: Churchill Livingstone Elsevier; 2006.

17. Iwama M. Open plenary speech to the College of Occupational Therapists Annual Conference 2013 [video file]. June 18, 2013. https://www.youtube.com/watch?v=67PqinQ7qNM. Accessed May 15, 2018.

18. Hammell KW. Sacred texts: a sceptical exploration of the assumptions underpinning theories of occupation. *Can J Occup Ther*. 2009;76(1):6-13.

19. Hammell KW. Resisting theoretical imperialism in the disciplines of occupational science and occupational therapy. *Br J Occup Ther*. 2011;74(1):27-33.

20. Yerxa E. Occupational terminology interactive dialogue. *J Occup Sci*. 1999;6:75-79.

21. Wilcock A, Townsend E. Occupational justice: occupational terminology interactive dialogue. *J Occup Sci*. 2000;7:84-86.

22. Wilcock A, Hocking C. *An Occupational Perspective of Health*. 3rd ed. Thorofare, NY: Slack Inc; 2015.

23. Pierce D. Promise. *J Occup Sci*. 2012;19(4):298-311.

24. American Occupational Therapy Association. Occupational therapy practice framework: domain and process. *Am J Occup Ther*. 2002;56:609-639.

25. American Occupational Therapy Association. Occupational therapy practice framework: domain and process, 3rd ed. *Am J Occup Ther*. 2014;68(suppl 1):S1-S48.

26. Kielhofner G. Respecting both the "occupation" and the "therapy" in our field. *Am J Occup Ther*. 2007;61:479-482.

27. Kielhofner G. *Model of Human Occupation: Theory and Application*. 4th ed. Baltimore, MD: Lippincott Williams & Wilkins; 2008.

28. Holmes W, Scaffa M. The nature of emerging practice in occupational therapy: a pilot study. *Occup Ther Health Care*. 2009;23(3):189-206.

29. Muñoz J, Dix S, Reichenbach D. Building productive roles: occupational therapy in a homeless shelter. *Occup Ther Health Care*. 2006;20(3/4):167-187.

30. Muir S. Occupational therapy in primary health care: we should be there. *Am J Occup Ther*. 2012;66(5):506-510.

31. Blakeney AB, Marshall A. Water quality, health, and human occupations. *Am J Occup Ther*. 2009;63(1):46-57.

32. Gupta J, Sullivan C. The central role of occupation in the doing, being and belonging of immigrant women. *J Occup Sci*. 2013;20(1):23-35.

33. American Occupational Therapy Association. *Salary and Workforce Survey*. Bethesda, MD: AOTA Press; 2015.

34. Reed KL, Peters CO. Occupational therapy: values and beliefs. The formative years 1904-1929. April 17, 2006. http://www.aota.org/publications-news/otp/values.aspx. Accessed May 15, 2018.

35. Reed K. *Models of Practice in Occupational Therapy*. Baltimore, MD: Lippincott Williams & Wilkins; 1984.

13 Ethics and a Changing Vision

In the history of our discipline there is probably no more important policy decision than this one, which changes the focus of service from patient to client.

—Mary Reilly[1]

American Journal of Occupational Therapy

Chapter Outline

A Changing Vision
  Issues With Client-Based Ethics
  Defining Value
Scope of Practice
  Provision of OT Services

Learning Objectives

1. Explain the purpose of the American Occupational Therapy Association *Vision 2025* document.
2. Describe the historic *patient* versus *client* debate and how it relates to contemporary practice.
3. Differentiate between the ethical systems that affect the definition and practice of occupational therapy in the United States.
4. Define *scope of practice* and outline the key tasks legally performed by occupational therapists in your state or region.

Key Terms

client-based ethics
patient-based ethics
scope of practice

Overview

The occupational therapy (OT) profession has experienced ongoing evolution of its theory base. We have seen in earlier chapters that the applied field of OT and the discipline of occupational science are still working out how they influence and support each other. The increasing globalization of the profession makes it apparent that different configurations of health care delivery systems have a large impact on the way that OT professionals provide care. We have learned that the practice of OT differs from country to country.

As our profession evolves, it is important for researchers and clinicians to accept and respond to critical dialogue. In her famous 1961 Slagle lecture,[2] Reilly describes the importance of criticism and public debate in professions. She stated:

> ... a card-carrying critic must do more than merely engage in critical thinking. Judgments made by a critic must emerge from a discreet use of techniques which are difficult to master and dangerous to apply. Basically, the skill is dependent upon an ability to analyze, interpret and synthesize. A critic must have a sharply developed capacity to see deficiencies in data and fallacies in interpretation. The best stock in trade that any critic has is a discerning eye for trends and an ability to pattern and verbalize them. Whether a critic is worth listening to is usually decided by an ability to use language well, by a creativeness in synthesizing new relations, and by courage to propose provocative hypotheses. Ultimately, however, a good critic rests his case upon how well he has been able to restructure the issue so that the necessary powers for its resolution can be freed.

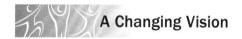 ## A Changing Vision

In 2017, the American Occupational Therapy Association (AOTA) released its *Vision 2025* document, which aims to guide the profession into the next decade. Its opening statement is "Occupational therapy maximizes health, well-being, and quality of life for all people, populations, and communities through effective solutions that facilitate participation in everyday living."[3] This vision statement followed the redefinitions of OT that occurred through several revisions of the Practice Framework (see Chapter 12). A notable change in both the Framework definition and the new vision statement is an increasing emphasis on population-based interventions.

Thirty years ago, an important philosophical debate arose in the profession centered on whether the term *patient* or *client* was more appropriate for OT. Reilly[1] argued that a move away from the term *patient* would equate to abandoning the moral base of the profession. She considered the change as abandonment of ethics around patient care, and without those ethics, the OT profession has to focus on contractually serving the needs of government and private agencies and insurance payers.

Yerxa and Sharrott[4] were also deeply concerned about abandoning **patient-based ethics**. They outlined several problems with **client-based ethics**, including that requests for medical care would be allotted on a preemptory basis and that the patient–health professional relationship would forfeit its compassion and trust for the adversarial relationship of legal ethics. They stated, "This could result in a normative, restrictive view of health, which robs patients of their liberty. The patient's role in developing goals pertinent to his or her concerns—and not necessarily consistent with those generated by health practitioners—could be adversely affected."

The OT profession may now be struggling with issues that were debated three decades ago. In addition to changes in the definition of OT, and the addition of population-based language to the current vision statement, the concept of social justice (also termed distributive justice) was recently included in the Code of Ethics as an enforceable principle.[5] Occupational therapists were instructed to advocate for the highest principles of social justice, but there was no clear definition of what social justice means in the context of practice. Some academicians have promoted a change to rights-based ethics on the basis of a new morality of resource distribution. Autonomy is simply lost in this new ethic, as pointed out by Durocher et al.[6]

Issues With Client-Based Ethics

Recent articles in the *American Journal of Occupational Therapy*[7] endorse the Institute for Healthcare Improvement's Triple Aim (see Chapter 10) of "improving the individual experience of care; improving the health of populations; and reducing the per capita costs of care for populations."[8] In endorsing this model, a new duty of occupational therapists is to control for costs that government and private payers are incurring for health care. Responsible therapists should always be economically prudent and should be properly cognizant of the costs associated with their services, but is it the primary role of occupational therapists to meet the economic objectives of government and private payers?

In pediatric practice, occupational therapists are now encouraged to provide services to school systems instead of children, and the professional association promulgates resource allocation and staffing on the basis of workload instead of a caseload.[9] *Caseload* refers to the number of students assigned to an occupational therapist, without regard for the amount of time needed to meet each student's needs or the therapist's other responsibilities within the broader school setting. *Workload* refers to all activities required to be performed by the occupational therapist and addresses the full range of demands on the professional's time. In this new configuration, the emphasis is transferred from the individual student to the larger system under which the individual is receiving services.

As another example, therapists are encouraged to consider marketing their services on the basis of how much money might be saved by preventing hospital readmissions.[10] These examples demonstrate the shift away from patient-based ethics in service to entities that govern the educational and health care payment systems.

If part of the purpose of OT is to play a role in "reducing the per capita costs of care for populations," then how does that position the profession ethically when it comes time to deliver care?

Defining Value

Government and private payers define *value* in terms of dollars spent. Most occupational therapists define *value* in terms of people helped (Figures 13-1 through 13-3). These are not mutually exclusive objectives, but aligning a professional purpose with cost-saving methodologies changes an entire ethical system. How is a therapist supposed to meet the occupational needs of his or her patients while at the same time meeting the economic and/or social justice objectives of organizational patrons?

It may be possible to achieve both goals, but doing so becomes increasingly challenging when government and private payment systems are defining *quality* in OT practice and basing it on economic or public health terms. A different set of ethics is required when working with patients as opposed to working in the interest of an organizational patron. One approach values autonomy and individual choice. The other focuses on the public good (including its economic good).

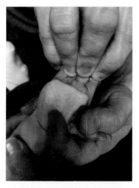

Figure 13-1   An occupational therapist applies an elastomer mold to a child's palm to reduce scarring from a burn. Courtesy of ABC Therapeutics.

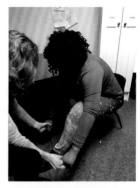

Figure 13-2   An occupational therapist helps a young child develop dressing skills. Courtesy of ABC Therapeutics.

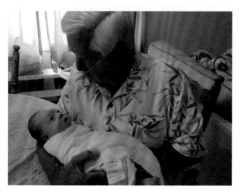

Figure 13-3   Energy conservation techniques suggested by an occupational therapist help a great-grandparent with chronic obstructive pulmonary disease participate in a caregiving role. Courtesy of ABC Therapeutics.

Occupational therapists have been warned that public health models are incompatible with OT.[11] Specifically, Reed suggests that "occupational therapists must be careful to differentiate between the public health model and the health education and wellness model." Braveman[12] asks, "How can we demonstrate occupational therapy's distinct value in improving the individual experience of care, improving the health of populations, and reducing the per capita cost of care?"

The problem of conflicting goals associated with patient- and client-based ethics that was raised 30 years ago continues to be a source of confusion in the evolving OT profession. This problem will need to be resolved for the profession to move forward.

Scope of Practice

In health care professions, **scope of practice** is a legal term used to describe the actions, procedures, and processes that a practitioner can engage in according to the terms of his or her professional license. In the United States, the practice of OT is specifically defined and regulated via state licensing laws.

Some more expansive definitions of OT, such as consultation to systems, management, program design, and education, are not frequently described as part of the OT scope of practice in state regulations. You do not need to be an occupational therapist to engage in many of these tasks. Failing to distinguish between what constitutes the *practice* of OT and tasks that an occupational therapist might do (on the basis of their knowledge and skills) contributes to an ongoing identity crisis. Many states primarily define OT around the treatment of individuals. The word *client* may be used, but it generally refers to individuals as clients, and regulations are oriented around *client factors* that are typically addressed. In addition, in most cases, practice requires the involvement of the doctor to provide referrals.

The newer definition of *client* encompasses individuals, institutions, communities, and populations. There is a steady stream of incrementalism in professional documents that continues to drift away from our philosophical core of direct patient service. Most state practice acts do not support the notion that therapists are licensed to solve the occupational problems of entire communities and populations, and yet these ideas are increasingly referenced in association documents and the professional literature.

In all professions, there are ancillary activities that professionals may engage in that do not precisely represent *practice* of the profession. Many of those activities draw upon the professional's related knowledge. However, because those activities might reasonably be completed by people with many different skill sets and types of professional training, engaging in those tasks cannot be considered a unique scope of practice for a single discipline.

When an occupational therapist designs an accessible playground (Figure 13-4), he or she may be using OT skills but are not practicing OT because many other professionals may also serve that same function. This fact does not make designing accessible playgrounds an unimportant task. However, if the OT profession seeks to survive in the health care arena, it needs to begin distinguishing between what actual *therapy* is and the "use of OT skills in related tasks."

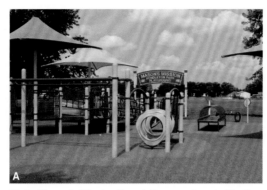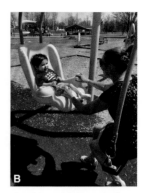

Figure 13-4   Mason's Mission Foundation was founded by the parents of two children who have disabilities. The parents' goal was to create fun and engaging opportunities for their children to play and where no child would feel any different than other children. In a full community effort that involved many different people and organizations, this group was able to create an all-inclusive, ADA-approved playground for the Western New York region. Photos courtesy of Mason's Mission Foundation and the Evchich Family. ADA, Americans with Disabilities Act.

This kind of systems consultation, or service to populations, does not represent a unique practice role for occupational therapists. That does not diminish the importance of these tasks. It just does not make them unique to the OT profession.

When there is conflation between the profession of OT and the ancillary good things that a therapist might do with his or her skills, the public's understanding of the profession may become less clear. This threatens reimbursement and creates unnecessary resource drain and potential legal challenge. It is arguable that the practice of occupational therapists, as they are employed under that title in their professional capacities, best represents the actual definition of OT.

Provision of OT Services

The National Board for Certification in Occupational Therapy (NBCOT) periodically conducts practice analysis studies to determine the domains, tasks, and knowledge needed to effectively practice to ensure that the certification exam reflects current practice. These analyses provide useful information regarding the tasks engaged in by new practitioners. There should be high levels of congruence between OT students' education and the tasks those students perform once they are in the field.

Dunn and Cada[13] reported the results of the 1998 NBCOT analysis of more than 3000 practitioners and identified population-based services as a practice area of new emphasis. Population-based services were rated at a low frequency of 4% to 5%, but this was adequate frequency to be included in the analysis report.

In the 2008 Practice Analysis,[14] services to populations were no longer a separate domain as it did not reach the level of frequency reported in the previous analysis. Services to populations had diminished frequency and were reflected only as an isolated point of knowledge, underneath the larger domain of "Selecting and implementing evidence based interventions." Accordingly, a much smaller percentage of items on the exam reflected this area.

The most recent practice analysis[15] surveyed nearly 3000 practitioners and again showed very low frequency for population-based services. Such services are reflected at the task and knowledge level related to overall program development and advocacy. There was not a high enough frequency to list this at a domain level.

Frequency of task engagement is a functional metric that should be used by the profession in defining its activities and scope of practice. Service to populations or whole communities is a low-frequency activity that does not represent a common area of OT practice in the United States. On the basis of evidence of validated tasks completed by practicing therapists, direct patient care remains at the core of professional responsibilities for U.S. practitioners and is also represented in domain-of-practice statements that are part of most licensing regulations.

Summary

- As the OT profession evolves, it is important for researchers and clinicians to accept and respond to critical dialogue.

- In 2017, the AOTA released its *Vision 2025* document, which aims to guide the profession into the next decade.

- Patient-based ethics are centered around patient care, whereas client-centered ethics may also require serving the needs and requirements of government and private agencies that pay for OT services.

- A different set of ethics is required when working with patients as opposed to working in the interest of an organizational patron. The patient-centered approach values autonomy and individual choice. The other focuses on the public good (including its economic good).

- *Scope of practice* is a legal term used to describe the actions, procedures, and processes that a health care practitioner can engage in according to the terms of his or her professional license. In the United States, the practice of OT is defined and regulated via state licensing laws.

- As a profession grows and evolves its service, it is important that new concepts be tested in the context of existing philosophy, theory, and legal definitions.

Reflect and Apply

Individual activity

1. Look up the scope of practice of OT as defined in your state licensing laws. Create a listing of specific services that are protected by your state and can be performed only by a licensed OT practitioner.

Class discussion

1. Read and critique the AOTA *Vision 2025* statement, including supporting and opposing opinions on the key phrases. Engage in a class debate about the power of the statement and ways that it might be improved.

2. Consider the following activities and engage in a class discussion about which type of professional might claim that he or she is best suited to these tasks. If multiple professionals might make claim to these activities, can they be legally protected as the scope of practice of any single profession? What are the implications of this dynamic for professions?
   a. Consulting to planners on Americans with Disabilities Act (ADA) requirement for bathroom accessibility in a new office complex
   b. Leading a community group that investigates universal design elements in a playground
   c. Developing a falls prevention program and presenting to a senior citizen group
   d. Promoting a clubhouse model when developing a community mental health program
   e. Providing a bullying awareness program in an elementary school
   f. Advocating at a city council meeting for curb cuts in a downtown shopping area
   g. Participating on a design team in developing powered mobility devices for toddlers
   h. Raising awareness of human sex trafficking and suggesting alternate policing strategies
   i. Developing a fitness event for parents and children in a local Head Start program
   j. Writing a grant to obtain funding for library materials for people with visual impairments

Review Questions

1. The purpose of the AOTA vision statement is to

   a. guide the association's strategic priorities.
   b. establish guidelines for insurance reimbursement.
   c. explain the purpose of the association.
   d. promote the OT profession.

2. In the patient–client debate, Reilly argued that

   a. the use of the word *client* was sometimes appropriate.
   b. the use of the word *client* meant abandoning the moral base of the profession.
   c. client-centered practice was the most ethical form for the OT profession.
   d. occupational therapists should adopt legal-based ethics in client care.

3. One concern expressed about client-based ethics was that

    a. OT services could be delivered only under contract.
    b. therapists would no longer be able to work in hospital settings.
    c. therapists would no longer be able to work in educational settings.
    d. the adversarial relationship of legal ethics would impact OT practice.

4. Which of the following principles was included in the AOTA Code of Ethics for the first time in 2010?

    a. Social justice
    b. Beneficence
    c. Fidelity
    d. Nonmaleficence

5. *Scope of practice* is defined as

    a. the philosophical perspective of a professional association.
    b. valuable activities that any licensed professional might engage in.
    c. the legal activities that the public can expect from a licensed professional.
    d. the evidence-based intervention techniques of any profession.

6. A survey used to determine the actual tasks performed regularly by entry-level practitioners is the

    a. AOTA Workforce Study.
    b. NBCOT Practice Analysis.
    c. Accreditation Council for Occupational Therapy Education (ACOTE) Standards.
    d. state licensing law.

7. Studies completed by NBCOT have clearly indicated that population-based services are

    a. infrequently provided by entry-level practitioners.
    b. increasingly being provided by entry-level practitioners.
    c. important for the OT profession to research.
    d. necessary for improving the relevance of OT practice.

8. In the United States, most OT practice is oriented around

    a. consultation to systems.
    b. cost-saving initiatives.
    c. grant writing and research.
    d. direct patient care.

References

1. Reilly M. The importance of the client vs. patient issue for occupational therapy. *Am J Occup Ther*. 1984;38(6):404-406.
2. Reilly M. Occupational therapy can be one of the greatest ideas of 20th century medicine. 1961 Eleanor Clarke Slagle Lecture. *Am J Occup Ther*. 1962;16:1-9.
3. American Occupational Therapy Association. Vision 2025. *Am J Occup Ther*. 2017;71(3):7103420010p1. doi:10.5014/ajot.2017.713002.
4. Yerxa EJ, Sharrott GW. Promises to keep: implications of the referent "patient" versus "client" for those served by occupational therapy. *Am J Occup Ther*. 1985;39(6):401-405.
5. Slater DY, ed. *Reference Guide to the Occupational Therapy Code of Ethics and Ethics Standards*. Bethesda, MD: AOTA Press; 2011.
6. Durocher E, Rappolt S, Gibson BE. Occupational justice: future directions. *J Occup Sci*. 2014;21(4):431-442.
7. Leland NE, Crum K, Phipps S, Roberts P, Gage B. Advancing the value and quality of occupational therapy in health service delivery. *Am J Occup Ther*. 2015;69(1):6901090010p1-6901090010p7. doi:10.5014/ajot.2015.691001.
8. Berwick DM, Nolan TW, Whittington J. The triple aim: care, health, and cost. *Health Affairs*. 2008;27:759-769. doi:10.1377/hlthaff.27.3.759.
9. American Occupational Therapy Association, American Physical Therapy Association, American Speech-Language Hearing Association. Workload approach: a paradigm shift for positive impact on student outcomes. 2014. http://www.aota.org/-/media/Corporate/Files/Practice/Children/APTA-ASHA-AOTA-Joint-Doc-Workload-Approach-Schools-2014.pdf. Accessed May 15, 2018.
10. Rogers AT, Bai G, Lavin RA, Anderson GF. Higher hospital spending on occupational therapy is associated with lower readmission rates. *Med Care Res Rev*. 2017;1-19. doi:10.1177/1077558716666981.
11. Reed KL. *Models of Practice in Occupational Therapy*. Baltimore, MD: Lippincott Williams & Wilkins; 1984.
12. Braveman B. Population health and occupational therapy. *Am J Occup Ther*. 2015;70:1-6.
13. Dunn W, Cada E. The national occupational therapy practice analysis: findings and implications for competence. *Am J Occup Ther*. 1998;52:721-728.
14. National Board for Certification in Occupational Therapy. Executive summary for the practice analysis study. Registered Occupational Therapist OTR®. 2008. http://www.nbcot.org. Accessed May 15, 2018.
15. National Board for Certification in Occupational Therapy. Practice analysis of the occupational therapist registered OTR®. 2012. http://www.nbcot.org. Accessed May 15, 2018.

Glossary

A

adaptation/compensation Modifying a task or environment to support occupational performance.

adaptive responses Successful and goal-directed actions that meet environmental demands.

applied science Use and study of acquired knowledge to solve practical problems.

attractor state Preferred movement patterns that represent stable efficiency states in which motor patterns tend to establish themselves based on system constraints.

autonomy Independence or freedom of action; the right of an individual to self-determination, privacy, confidentiality, and consent.

B

backward chaining Method used in applied behavior analysis in which a task is broken down into component steps. All the behaviors in a single task are completed by the trainer except the last step that the individual is attempting to master.

basic science Study/research conducted with the goal of basic scientific discovery.

beneficence Action done for the benefit of others.

biomechanical model Model of practice that focuses primarily on physical structures of the body and their efficiency and function for movement.

biomedical Related to addressing physical and mental/emotional impairments and problems.

biosocial Interaction or combination of biologic and social factors.

C

cardiovascular endurance Refers to the ability of the circulatory and respiratory systems to deliver oxygenated blood to all body systems to meet metabolic demands.

case formulation In the neurofunctional approach, a story that is used to create a shared understanding of the situation.

client-based ethics A legalistic and rights-based system for directing health care decisions and services.

closed system System that has little or no interaction with other systems or the environment.

cognition Mental processes involved in perception, thinking, reasoning, learning, and memory.

cognitive disability model Practice model focused on the concept of functional cognition.

cognitive orientation to daily occupational performance (CO-OP) model Practice model focused on a performance-based and problem-solving approach to cognitive skill acquisition.

cognitive rehabilitation model Practice model focused on development of information processing skills needed for occupational performance.

constraint-induced movement therapy (CIMT) Method of restraining an unimpaired extremity to restrict use of the stronger extremity and force the patient to use the impaired extremity.

D

dynamic interactional model Practice model focused on a restorative and systems-level approach to improving occupational performance.

dynamometer Assessment device used to measure muscle power.

E

eclecticism An approach based on choosing aspects from multiple theories, concepts, or practices.

ecology of human performance (EHP) model Occupation-based model developed because of a need to emphasize contextual elements such as temporality, environment, and other external factors that can impact occupational performance.

educational standards Set of requirements for what students must be taught in a specific academic program.

egalitarianism Belief that all people are equal and deserving of equal rights and opportunities.

emergence The occurrence of complex motor actions that result from the interaction of the person, the task requirements, and the environment.

ethics Moral principles that govern the behavior of an individual or the actions of an organization.

ethnography Scientific description of societies and cultures; a branch of anthropology that involves studying people in a particular society or culture by observing them in their natural setting.

F

fidelity Degree to which an intervention is implemented according to its underlying theoretical principles and procedural guidelines.

forward chaining Method used in applied behavior analysis in which a task is broken down into component steps. The individual is provided reinforcement for successfully completing individual steps occurring in a sequence to form a complex behavior.

founders Individuals who create a new enterprise.

functional cognition In the cognitive disability model, refers to dynamic interaction between the individual's cognitive abilities and activities or performance contexts.

functional movement Movement required to engage in daily occupations.

G

general systems theory The premise that a system is made up of parts that interact to form a coherent whole and that complex systems share organizing principles.

globalization The spread of ideas, goods, services, and technologies around the world.

goniometer Assessment device used to measure range of motion in a joint.

H

habit training Treatment methodology developed by Slagle whereby patients were provided with round-the-clock supervision for participating in everyday routines.

habituation Process of organizing actions into patterns and routines of performance.

hierarchical control Traditional theory of motor control stating that higher-level cortical centers exert command and control over lower-level midbrain and brain stem levels.

hierarchy A ranking system that places elements one above the other.

I

imperialism Extension of influence, power, and/or dominion from one country or region to another, often by force.

implementation science Study of methods to promote the integration of research findings and evidence into health care policy and practice.

J

justice Condition of being morally correct or fair.

L

learned nonuse Self-reinforcing negative attractor state that occurs when a person with a weaker extremity uses the stronger extremity to perform tasks because it is easier to do so.

M

maintenance Interventions designed to keep biomechanical performance at a specified level of functioning.

medical model Science-based methods used by occupational therapists that reflect the values and methods of physicians.

model A representation of a system or methodology based on a set of rules and concepts.

model of human occupation (MOHO) Practice model developed primarily by Kielhofner that was an expansion and clarification of the occupational behavior work done by Reilly and her students.

model of practice An approach and structure used to guide interventions.

moral treatment Philosophy that treatment of mental illness should be based on humane psychosocial principles.

motor control Process by which the brain controls and coordinates muscles to produce movement and accomplish task behavior.

motor function Movement or activity that occurs due to the activation of motor neurons.

motor learning The central nervous system's response to practice or experience when developing a new motor skill.

multicontext approach In the dynamic interactional model, a method that involves learning skills in multiple environments to support transfer of learning.

muscle tone The resting tension of a muscle.

muscular endurance Refers to the ability to sustain muscular activity over a specified period of time or to complete a specific task.

N

neurofunctional approach (NFA) Practice model designed for use when more severe deficits are present that is focused on improving cognitive function by training in specific tasks.

neuroplasticity The brain's ability to form and reorganize synaptic connections in response to experience.

NOBA method Reilly's concept stating that clinicians should *not only* focus on biomedical or reductionistic science *but also* remember to attend to biosocial concerns.

nonmaleficence Avoiding causing harm or inflicting the least harm possible to reach a beneficial outcome.

O

occupation Activities of daily living, including self-care, education, work, play, leisure, social participation, rest, and sleep.

occupational adaptation A normative process of occupation used by individuals to meet environmental demands.

occupational adaptation (OA) model Practice model focused on the interaction between the person and the environment to help individuals meet environmental demands.

occupational behavior model An incompletely articulated occupational therapy model developed by Reilly and her students in response to Reilly's call for a return to a focus on occupation.

occupational justice The right of every person to be able to meet basic needs and have equal opportunities to reach toward his/her potential that is specific to the individual's engagement in diverse and meaningful occupation.

occupational performance A person's ability to complete a task related to his/her self-care, productivity, or leisure participation.

occupational science Interdisciplinary field engaged in the study of humans as occupational beings.

occupational therapy Health care profession that uses occupations to promote health and wellness, to remediate or restore function, to maintain health, and to prevent disease and injury.

open system System that interacts with other systems and/or with the outside environment.

ordinary meaning Legal concept referring to the everyday definition and interpretation of a particular word, phrase, or idea.

orthotic External device or appliance that supports musculoskeletal function or positions a body part in a position of function or protection.

P

paradigm Broad perspective or a shared set of ideas across a particular group or profession.

paradigm crisis Occurs when questions emerge about the shared values and beliefs of a scientific community or a professional group.

paradigm of occupation The first philosophical construct of the occupational therapy profession, based on the belief that occupation should be used as a treatment modality.

paradigm shift A fundamental change in the basic concepts and practices of a profession.

patient-based ethics A morals-based system for directing health care decisions and services.

perceived self-efficacy A person's beliefs about his/her ability to perform.

performance capacity The physical and mental processes and abilities that underlie the performance of an activity.

person–environment–occupation (PEO) models Group of theoretical approaches that share common elements of focusing on the transactional relationship between the person, the environment, and the occupations being performed by an individual.

phenomenology The study of a person's subjective experience; branch of philosophy that deals with consciousness, thought, and experience.

philosophy Statements that outline the beliefs of a specific group of people; the theoretical basis of a profession.

population health The health outcomes of members of a population, including the distribution of such outcomes within the group.

postural control A person's ability to maintain their center of gravity over their base of support.

posture Position of the limbs or carriage of the body as a whole.

practice setting Location in which occupational therapy services are provided.

practice standards Set of guidelines and criteria for providing care.

praxis Neurologic process by which people plan and direct motor action and planning and executing a movement.

prevention Intervention strategy designed to avoid negative outcomes and to promote overall health and well-being.

proprioception The sense of where body parts are in space.

public health Actions taken by a society to collectively ensure the conditions in which people can be healthy.

R

range of motion The amount of movement possible at a joint.

reconstruction aides Civilian women who provided treatment in the form of physical and occupational therapy to assist in the rehabilitation of servicemen during and after World War I.

reductionism Analyzing and describing a complex phenomenon in terms of its component parts.

reflex Action or movement not controlled by conscious thought; occurs in response to a stimulus.

reflex arc Nerve pathway in a reflex that includes sensory and motor components.

release phenomenon Phenomenon that occurs when abnormal reflexive movement patterns controlled by lower-brain centers act without the inhibition of higher-brain control centers.

remediation/rehabilitation Restoration of function through targeted training based on evidence-based assessment and intervention planning.

rest cure Practice of using extended bed rest and inactivity as a treatment for illness or disease.

S

scope of practice Legal term used to describe the actions, procedures, and processes that a practitioner can engage in according to the terms of their professional license.

self-awareness In social cognitive theory, refers to an ability to understand one's own self and abilities in relation to the external environment.

sensory integration The organization of sensation for use.

sensory integration model Practice model designed to explain how the brain organizes sensory information to generate adaptive responses.

settlement house Facility in poor, urban areas established in the late 19th and early 20th centuries that provided living space and educational, recreational, and social services to alleviate poverty and other social ills.

social cognitive theory Psychological theory that states that people learn as a function of their environment and their own personal factors, but are still capable of self-reflection and self-regulation.

social justice The fair, equitable, and appropriate distribution of resources, rights, and responsibilities in society; also called *distributive justice.*

sociopolitical determinants of health Socioeconomic and political factors that influence the health status of individuals or populations.

strength The amount of available muscle power a person can activate to perform a movement or task.

T

tactile Related to the sense of touch.

task-oriented approach Training on specific functional motor tasks, developing practice schedules, and individualizing feedback to meet the needs of different learning styles.

theory Set of ideas intended to explain a phenomenon or serve as a set of principles on which some type of practice is based.

translational science Methodology of applying basic scientific findings to solve real-world problems.

Triple Aim An initiative of the Institute of Healthcare Improvement oriented toward improving the experience of care, improving the health of populations, and reducing per-capita costs of health care.

V

veracity Truthfulness or accuracy.

vestibular sense Sensory system related to body position, head orientation, posture, and motion.

volition MOHO concept that refers to the power to make a choice or decision that motivates human action.

W

whole-task method Training method that allows a learner to practice an entire task to completion.

work cure Process of engaging patients in useful activities and training them in new skills as part of recovery from illness or disease.

work hardening Systematized method of physical reconditioning and rehabilitation that helps injured workers return to their employment.

Index

Note: Page numbers followed by " f " denote figures; those followed by " t " denote tables.

CCS0818